C000003482

Treatment Strategy for Unexplained Infertility and Recurrent Miscarriage

Keiji Kuroda • Jan J. Brosens
Siobhan Quenby • Satoru Takeda
Editors

Treatment Strategy for Unexplained Infertility and Recurrent Miscarriage

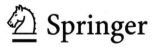 Springer

Editors
Keiji Kuroda
Center for Reproductive Medicine and
Implantation Research
Sugiyama Clinic Shinjuku
Tokyo
Japan

Department of Obstetrics and Gynaecology
Faculty of Medicine
Juntendo University
Tokyo
Japan

Siobhan Quenby
The Division of Biomedical Sciences
Clinical Science Research Laboratories
Warwick Medical School
Coventry
United Kingdom

Jan J. Brosens
The Division of Biomedical Sciences
Clinical Science Research Laboratories
Warwick Medical School
Coventry
United Kingdom

Satoru Takeda
Department of Obstetrics and Gynaecology
Juntendo University
Tokyo
Japan

ISBN 978-981-10-8689-2   ISBN 978-981-10-8690-8   (eBook)
https://doi.org/10.1007/978-981-10-8690-8

Library of Congress Control Number: 2018944474

© Springer Nature Singapore Pte Ltd. 2018
This work is subject to copyright. All rights are reserved by the Publisher, whether the whole or part of the material is concerned, specifically the rights of translation, reprinting, reuse of illustrations, recitation, broadcasting, reproduction on microfilms or in any other physical way, and transmission or information storage and retrieval, electronic adaptation, computer software, or by similar or dissimilar methodology now known or hereafter developed.
The use of general descriptive names, registered names, trademarks, service marks, etc. in this publication does not imply, even in the absence of a specific statement, that such names are exempt from the relevant protective laws and regulations and therefore free for general use.
The publisher, the authors and the editors are safe to assume that the advice and information in this book are believed to be true and accurate at the date of publication. Neither the publisher nor the authors or the editors give a warranty, express or implied, with respect to the material contained herein or for any errors or omissions that may have been made. The publisher remains neutral with regard to jurisdictional claims in published maps and institutional affiliations.

Printed on acid-free paper

This Springer imprint is published by the registered company Springer Nature Singapore Pte Ltd.
The registered company address is: 152 Beach Road, #21-01/04 Gateway East, Singapore 189721, Singapore

Preface

Since the world's first IVF baby was born in 1978, over a half-century ago, reproductive technologies including diagnosis and treatment of reproductive disorders have been significantly advanced. In 1990–1992, the first babies after human embryo vitrification and intracytoplasmic injection were born; then it seemed as if all infertility causes would be overcome.

It is estimated that more than seven million babies have been born by IVF; however, its success rate is still 20–30% per cycle of oocyte retrieval. In several countries, preimplantation genetic screening (PGS), which is embryo chromosomal testing, has been increasingly common, yet the success rate of IVF after PGS is less than 70% per embryo transfer; therefore more than 30% of unsuccessful causes of IVF are not derived from embryos. Also, recurrent miscarriage (RM) also remains unexplained in more than 50% of the women. As regarding humans, the rate of embryo wastage and pregnancy loss is quite high among the animal kingdom. Thus, the patients with unexplained RM may not achieve delivery by coincidence, but pregnancy losses may result from undetectable factors. As a result, gynaecologists often repeatedly provide these couples with general treatments for infertility and miscarriage or even discontinue treatment because they cannot detect the reason, which places serious financial, physical and mental burdens on the couples affected.

Unknown causes of reproductive failure have been revealed via mutual interaction between clinical medicine and basic research. We hope that this book will provide partial solution to unsolved factors of reproductive failure in the future.

Tokyo, Japan   Keiji Kuroda
Tokyo, Japan   Satoru Takeda

Contents

Part I
Unexplained Infertility

Chapter 1
Unexplained Infertility: Introduction

Keiji Kuroda

Abstract Among infertile couples, 15–30% are diagnosed with unexplained infertility after basic fertility tests. These couples cannot achieve a pregnancy due to accident or to undetected causes, including (1) oviduct dysfunction with tubal patency, (2) fertilization failure and (3) implantation failure without an organic lesion. If the duration of infertility is 2 years or longer, the patients have a high likelihood of an undetectable infertility factor. It is difficult to unsolve the reasons for infertility by timed intercourse or intrauterine insemination. Therefore, active infertility treatment, including in vitro fertilization, should be recommended.

Keywords Unexplained infertility · Tubal dysfunction · Fertilization failure · Implantation failure · In vitro fertilization

In humans, pregnancy requires achievement of various processes, such as encounter of the sperm and egg, fertilization, embryo development and implantation of a competent embryo to a receptive decidualized endometrium. Fertility can be assessed by monthly fecundity rate, that is, the probability of achieving pregnancy within one menstrual cycle. Compared to other mammalian species, the average human monthly fecundity rate is extremely low at 20%. Therefore, the potential cumulative pregnancy rate for normally fertile couples is 70–80%, 90–95% and 100% at 6, 12 and 24 months, respectively [1]. Infertility, in one in seven couples, is defined as inability to achieve a pregnancy after 1 year of regular unprotected intercourse. The causes of infertility are varied, including abnormality of sperm findings, ovulation disorder, fallopian tube occlusion or damage and endometriosis (Fig. 1.1). Unexplained infertility is diagnosed as the finding of no specific cause of infertility in approximately 15–30% of these couples after general fertility examinations, including hysterosalpingography, confirmation of ovulation, serum anti-Müllerian hormone level as ovarian reserve, postcoital testing and sperm testing [2, 3]. Female

K. Kuroda
Center for Reproductive Medicine and Implantation Research, Sugiyama Clinic Shinjuku, Tokyo, Japan

Department of Obstetrics and Gynaecology, Faculty of Medicine, Juntendo University, Tokyo, Japan
e-mail: arthur@juntendo.ac.jp

© Springer Nature Singapore Pte Ltd. 2018
K. Kuroda et al. (eds.), *Treatment Strategy for Unexplained Infertility and Recurrent Miscarriage*, https://doi.org/10.1007/978-981-10-8690-8_1

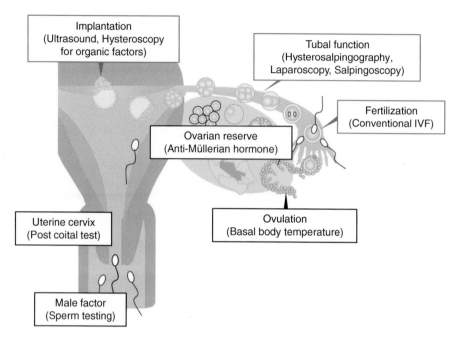

Fig. 1.1 Causes of infertility and examinations performed for the causes. It is difficult to assess tubal function of gamete and embryo transport and oocyte retrieval, fertilization and implantation using basic fertility tests (causes of infertility in red flame)

fecundity decreases with increasing age. Thus, some infertile women of late reproductive age may not conceive fortuitously, but patients with unexplained infertility cannot achieve pregnancy due to undetected causes of infertility after basic fertility tests have been performed [4]. The possible undetected causes of infertility are spermatozoa entrance failure at the uterotubal junction, tubal disorder of gamete and embryo transport, tube fimbria dysfunction of oocyte retrieval, fertilization failure, developmental disturbance of embryos and implantation failure (Fig. 1.2). At any rate, patients with unexplained infertility cannot conceive because of the undetectable causes affecting the processes of sperm-egg encounter or implantation between the embryo and the decidualized endometrium. Thus, they cannot benefit much from general infertility treatment, including timed intercourse or intrauterine insemination (IUI).

If a woman with unexplained infertility is young and cannot achieve pregnancy for 2 years or less, she may not achieve pregnancy accidentally. Therefore, National Institute for Health and Clinical Excellence (NICE) guidelines recommend general infertility treatment. If the duration of infertility is 2 years or longer, the patients have a high likelihood of an undetectable infertility factor. The reasons for infertility are unresolved by timed intercourse or IUI. Therefore, NICE guidelines recommend assisted reproductive technology (ART), including in vitro fertilization [2]. Gynaecologists should not repeat timed intercourse or IUI discursively during infertility treatment in patients without detectable causes of infertility. They should offer

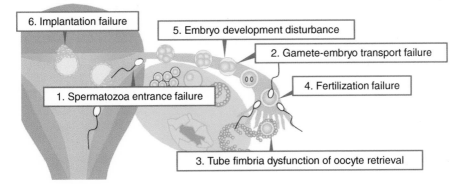

6. Implantation failure

5. Embryo development disturbance

2. Gamete-embryo transport failure

4. Fertilization failure

1. Spermatozoa entrance failure

3. Tube fimbria dysfunction of oocyte retrieval

Fig. 1.2 Candidate causes in patients with unexplained infertility. Unexplained infertility is defined as an unsuccessful pregnancy due to causes that are undetected by general fertility tests. Candidate causes of infertility are spermatozoa entrance failure at the uterotubal junction, gamete and embryo transport failure, tube fimbria dysfunction of oocyte retrieval, fertilization failure, developmental disturbance of embryos and implantation failure

an explanation why the patients cannot conceive and discuss active infertility treatment, including ART. The causes of unexplained infertility often are found during ART treatment.

Some cases of unexplained infertility are intractable even if the couples proceed to ART. We demonstrated unexplained infertility due to three factors in this book: (1) oviduct dysfunction with tubal patency, (2) fertilization failure and (3) implantation failure without an organic lesion. We hope the all readers will enhance their understanding of the knowledge of unexplained infertility and offer optimal infertility treatment.

References

1. Evers JLH. Female subfertility. Lancet. 2002;360:151–9.
2. NICE. National Institute for Health and Clinical Excellence. National Collaborating Centre for Women's and Children's Health. Fertility: Assessment and Treatment for People with Fertility Problems 2013;156:63.
3. Practice Comm Amer Soc Reprod M. Effectiveness and treatment for unexplained infertility. Fertil Steril. 2006;86:S111–4.
4. Somigliana EPA, Busnelli A, Filippi F, Pagliardini L, Vigano P, Vercellini P. Age-related infertility and unexplained infertility: an intricate clinical dilemma. Hum Reprod. 2016;31:1390–6.

Chapter 2
Fertilization Failure

Takashi Yamaguchi, Keiji Kuroda, Atsushi Tanaka, and Seiji Watanabe

Abstract The early stage of fertilization is the cell fusion of the sperm and the egg, which in a narrow sense is the definition of fertilization. In unfertilized eggs, meiosis is stopped at a species-specific stage. The early stage of fertilization breaks the pause in the cell division and meiosis resumes. This is called oocyte activation; this activation allows meiosis to be completed, and the male and female pronuclei are then formed. The fusion of the male and female genomes (syngamy) completes the fertilization in the broad sense. On the other hand, fertilization is not established if the fertility of the eggs or sperm is impaired. The improvement of fertilization rates by micro insemination (intracytoplasmic sperm injection, ICSI) is remarkable. However, there are many cases in which fertilization is not achieved even after ICSI. In such severe infertility cases, the artificial activation of the oocyte is one possible solution. Therefore, we examined the effectiveness of various ovum activation methods from both aspects of cytological evaluation (embryogenesis) and biochemical evaluation (intracellular Ca^{2+} responses).

Keywords Fertilization failure · Human oocyte · Egg activation · Phospholipase C zeta (PLCζ) · Ca^{2+} oscillations · Intracytoplasmic sperm injection · Assisted oocyte activation

T. Yamaguchi
Department of Obstetrics and Gynaecology, Faculty of Medicine, Juntendo University, Tokyo, Japan

Saint Mother Obstetrics and Gynecology Clinic, Institute for ART, Fukuoka, Japan

K. Kuroda (✉)
Department of Obstetrics and Gynaecology, Faculty of Medicine, Juntendo University, Tokyo, Japan

Center for Reproductive Medicine and Implantation Research, Sugiyama Clinic Shinjuku, Tokyo, Japan
e-mail: arthur@juntendo.ac.jp

A. Tanaka
Saint Mother Obstetrics and Gynecology Clinic, Institute for ART, Fukuoka, Japan

S. Watanabe
Department of Anatomical Science, Hirosaki University Graduate school of Medicine, Aomori, Japan

© Springer Nature Singapore Pte Ltd. 2018
K. Kuroda et al. (eds.), *Treatment Strategy for Unexplained Infertility and Recurrent Miscarriage*, https://doi.org/10.1007/978-981-10-8690-8_2

2.1   Introduction

Ovulated mature eggs are surrounded by zona pellucida and cumulus cell layers; meiosis is stopped at the second meiotic division until the penetration of the spermatozoa [1]. Spermatozoa reaching the egg pass through the hyaluronic acid substrate surrounding the egg and bind to the zona pellucida. Sperm that has passed through the zona pellucida fuses with the cell membrane of the ovum and is taken into the egg cytoplasm. Sperm penetration induces ovum surface response and meiosis reinitiation. In mature eggs, the surface granules containing the enzyme are distributed right under the cell membrane, and the surface layer granules are opened and secreted to the perivitelline space by the surface reaction. The released enzyme removes some sugar chains from the zona pellucida glycoprotein, causing protein denaturation. Then the binding and passage of the sperm to the zona pellucida are inhibited. Egg cell membranes also change, so that sperm cannot fuse. These changes are called the zona reaction and the cortical change of the egg and have the role of preventing multi-sperm fertilization [2].

On the other hand, fertilization is not established if the fertility of the eggs or sperm is impaired. The improvement of fertilization rates by micro insemination (intracytoplasmic sperm injection method, ICSI) is remarkable; however, there are many cases in which fertilization is not achieved even after ICSI [3]. There are cases in which the fertilization rate shows a value of 25% or less despite the quality of eggs being normal [4–6]. In such severe infertility cases, the artificial activation of the egg is one possible solution. Therefore, we examined the effectiveness of various oocyte activation methods from both aspects of cytological evaluation (embryogenesis) and biochemical evaluation (intracellular Ca^{2+} responses).

2.2   Fertilization Failure

Motility, capacitation, and acrosome reaction of human sperm are important events in the process of in vivo fertilization; however they are not essential when performing ICSI. The confirmation of the second polar body and the pronuclei indicates a probably successful fertilization. Even in the case of round spermatid cells and immature spermatogenic cells, fertilization has been confirmed when egg activation was artificially induced [7, 8].

The causes of the fertility disorder can be divided into cases derived from the gamete itself and the environment surrounding the gamete in vivo. The former is the number and quality of gametes, and the latter is a problem in the environment inside the female reproductive tract. When we consider the causes of the fertility disorders from the aspect of sperm, spermatogenesis, spermiogenesis, conditions inside the female reproductive organs, chemical composition of the tubal fluid surrounding cumulus cells, the interaction with the zona pellucida, membrane fusion, and egg activation are common problems. Whereas regarding egg cause infertility, egg reservation, oogenesis, egg nuclear, and cytoplasmic maturation, the nature of the zona pellucida, membrane fusion, ability to activate the egg itself resuming the second meiosis cooperating with a penetrating sperm, and the process leading to nuclear fusion are common problems.

Here we focus on what happens on the ICSI oocytes that fail to form pronuclei. From the sperm side, this phenomenon implies a lack or an insufficiency of sperm factor to initiate the egg activation. From the egg side, it means that egg activation depending on intracellular signaling triggered by sperm factors does not occur.

2.3 Treatment Strategy for Fertilization Failure

2.3.1 Intracytoplasmic Sperm Injection (ICSI)

In infertility treatment, one of the most powerful treatments for male factor and fertilization failure is the direct injection of a single sperm into the egg, this is known as ICSI. ICSI techniques are very advanced now, so fertilization rates are high, roughly 70–80% after ICSI [3]. However, no fertilized egg is recognized in 1–5% of ICSI cycles [9, 10]. This could be due to oocyte fertilization failure. To determine reasons of fertilization failure after ICSI, we have attempted a cytogenetic analysis of human ICSI oocytes in which no pronucleus was seen 12 h after insemination with the gradual fixation-air drying method.

Out of 92 ICSI oocytes examined, 84 (91.3%) remained at the meiotic metaphase II (MII), suggesting that oocyte activation had not yet happen even 12 h after ICSI (Fig. 2.1). Sperm nuclei found in the cytoplasm of the unactivated oocyte were classified into four types based on the degree of DNA decondensation (Fig. 2.1b–e). The first group consisted of the sperm heads with the plasma membrane surrounding the nucleus intact (Fig. 2.1a–c). Such sperm head nucleus was stained deep purple, and occasionally the sperm tail and acrosomal cap could be found. In these intact sperm, the remaining plasma membrane may prevent sperm factor to be released into the ooplasm. Therefore, there are cases when the sperm membrane is not digested in the ooplasm despite an application of the immobilization operation. In the other three groups, oocytes seem to be responsible for fertilization failure. The second group consists of the swollen heads, which have round-shaped swollen nucleus freed from the plasma membrane and were stained bright purple (Fig. 2.1d). This phenomenon results from dissociation of protamine disulfide bonds that allow sperm DNA to condense tightly. The third group includes a condensing chromatin mass (Fig. 2.1e). Cytostatic factor contained in the MII oocyte cytoplasm compels sperm DNA to condense into thin chromatin fibers replacing protamine with somatic histone. The prematurely condensed chromatin fibers generally appear to be thinner than the fibers replicated during S phase. The fourth group is made of prematurely condensed chromosomes (PCC), in which centromeres and chromosomal arms can be distinguished under a light microscope (Fig. 2.2). On the other hand, formation of pronucleus, which proves that the oocyte activation happens, was confirmed in

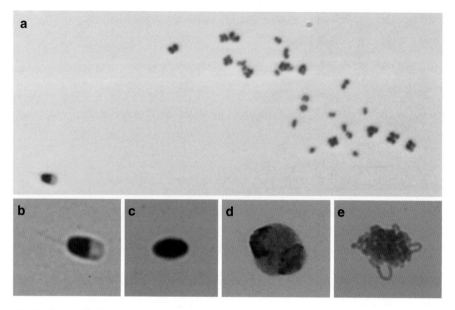

Fig. 2.1 Sperm heads found in underutilized ICSI oocytes that failed to form pronuclei at day 1. (**a**) Twenty-three meiotic chromosomes and a sperm with acrosome and tail (**b**) was found in a ICSI oocyte. (**c**) A sperm nucleus freed from the plasma membrane. (**d**) A swollen sperm nucleus. (**e**) A condensing chromatin mass (bar = 5 μm)

Fig. 2.2 Prematurely condensed chromosomes derived from sperm and oocyte meiotic chromosomes (×1000). Thin prematurely condensed chromatin of sperm (arrows) and oocyte chromosomes at the second meiotic metaphase, which consist of two homologous sister chromatids (arrow heads)

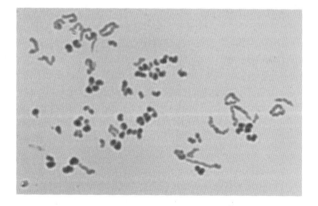

some oocytes after Giemsa staining, although it was not seen on a light microscope before preparation. In an oocyte with one pronucleus, a prematurely condensed chromatin mass which was presumptively derived from sperm nucleus was observed. Oocytes with large female pronucleus and small male pronucleus were also seen (Fig. 2.3). The results of the analysis are summarized in Table 2.1. The data shows that the main cause of fertilization failure in ICSI treatment is impaired oocyte activation. Hence these oocytes need some treatment to achieve fertilization.

Fig. 2.3 Two pronuclei fond in an unfertilized ICSI oocytes (×400). Large female and small male pronuclei were identified inside an oocyte after fixation and 2% Giemsa staining, although they were not confirmed under a light microscope

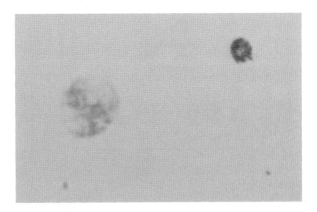

Table 2.1 The result of cytogenetic analysis in ICSI oocytes without microscopically visible pronucleus

	N	%
No. of oocytes analyzed	90	
No. of oocytes inactivated (meiotic metaphase II)	84	93.3
1. Intact sperm	12	13.3
2. Swollen head	7	7.8
3. Condensing chromatin	49	54.4
4. Prematurely condensed chromosomes	16	17.7
No. of oocytes activated	6	6.7

2.3.2 Assisted Oocyte Activation (AOA)

Sperm penetration induces Ca^{2+} oscillations, which is a repetitive transient rise in calcium ion concentration ($[Ca^{2+}]i$) in the egg. As shown in Fig. 2.4c, the ICSI procedure also induces a series of Ca^{2+} oscillations as conventional IVF. This rise allows the continuation of the meiosis after resumption of the second meiotic division. This phenomenon is called oocyte activation; the chromosome separates and shifts to the second meiotic anaphase and releases the second polar body, leading to formation of male and female pronuclei (PN) and cleavage of the embryo. Each Ca^{2+} oscillation results from Ca^{2+} release from the cellular endoplasmic reticulum through inositol 1,4,5-trisphosphate (IP3) receptor [11–14]. Ca^{2+} oscillations are induced by a cytosolic sperm factor at sperm-egg fusion [15]. Evidence indicates that a sperm-specific isozyme "zeta" of IP3-producing enzyme phospholipase C zeta (PLCζ) is a strong candidate as a sperm factor [12, 16–18]. PLCζ removal from sperm extract by anti-PLCζ antibody abolished the Ca^{2+} release in the eggs [16]. PLCζ RNA injection induced Ca^{2+} oscillations, which were indistinguishable from those at fertilization, and those at the egg activation, leading to development into blastocysts parthenogenetically [16, 19]. Injected recombinant PLCζ protein in the oocytes could elicit Ca^{2+} oscillations [20, 21]. Knockdown of PLCζ in transgenic mice resulted in low ability of egg activation with impaired Ca^{2+} oscillation and no offspring [22].

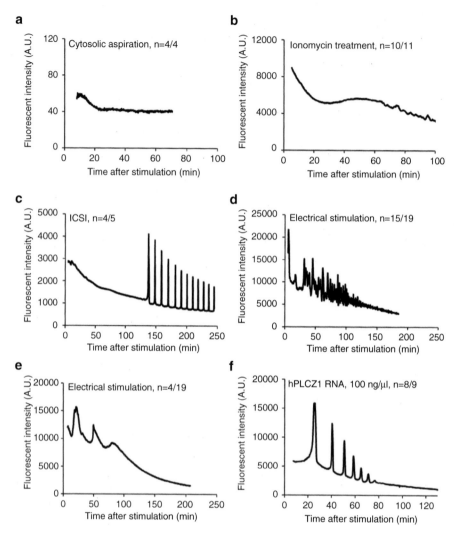

Fig. 2.4 Induction of Ca²⁺ responses in human oocyte by various active oocyte activation agents and procedures. Ca²⁺ responses in human oocyte induced by cytosolic aspiration (**a**), ionomycin treatment (**b**), ICSI (**c**), electrical stimulation (**d, e**), and human PLCZ1 (hPLCZ1) RNA (**f**, 100 ng/ μl). The timing of stimulation was set as the zero time. The numbers on each graph represent the number of oocytes displaying Ca²⁺ responses per total number of oocytes examined

Most cases of fertilization failure can be resolved by ICSI; however fertilization failure is observed in 1–5% of cases following ICSI [9, 10]. Then as in previous outcomes, main fertilization failure in ICSI treatment resulted from oocyte activation deficiency (Table 2.1). Assisted oocyte activation (AOA) can induce transient Ca²⁺ increase in the oocyte. AOA is an efficient procedure for couples with a history of low or failed fertilization after ICSI treatment. Various methods of AOA have been reported including mechanical, electrical, and chemical activation (Table 2.2).

Table 2.2 Assisted oocyte activation

Assisted oocyte activation	References
Mechanical activation	
(Cytosolic aspiration and injection)	Tesarik et al. [23]
Electrical activation	Yanagida et al. [24]
Chemical activation	
Strontium chloride	Kishikawa et al. [25]
Puromycin	Murase et al. [26]
6-DMAP	Szollosi et al. [27]
Phorbol esters	Cuthbertson and Cobbold [28]
Thimerosal	Fissore et al. [29]
Calcium ionophore	Steinhardt et al. [30]
Ionomycin	
Calcimycin (A23187)	

The popular assisted activation agents in human eggs as clinical applications include electrical pulses and calcium ionophores; however an established AOA has still not been determined.

Impaired function and abnormal form of sperm-specific egg-activating factor, PLCζ is associated with oocyte activation deficiency [31–34]. In a previous study, we evaluated the efficiency of several AOA methods for human oocyte activation including human PLCζ, hPLCZ1 RNA injection by measuring the $[Ca^{2+}]i$ responses [35].

2.3.2.1 Mechanical Activation

Tesarik et al. reported mechanical oocyte activation in 2002 as modified ICSI [23]. This mechanical AOA method aspirates ooplasm that is as close as possible to the oocyte periphery and reinject it in the center of the oocyte. Cytosolic aspiration and injection is repeated two to three times. The process consists of transferring Ca^{2+} in the oocyte periphery to the center of the oocyte. However, in 2004, Ebner et al. showed that modified ICSI did not improve fertilization, blastocyst formation, or clinical pregnancy rates after comparing data of conventional and modified ICSI in couples with a history of fertilization failure [36]. Our experiments also demonstrated that modified ICSI brought only a slight single Ca^{2+} rise which was completely different from physiological Ca^{2+} oscillations (Fig. 2.4a) [35].

2.3.2.2 Chemical Activation

Chemical agents for oocyte activation include strontium chloride [25], puromycin [26], 6-DMAP [27], phorbol esters [28], thimerosal [29], and calcium ionophore [30]. Calcium ionophores, such as ionomycin and calcimycin (A23187), are the most widespread AOA agents. Calcium ionophores can induce an influx of Ca^{2+} inside oocytes by going through the plasma membrane. Several reviews reported that the evidence of the effect of calcium ionophores is still insufficient, but calcium ionophores may improve fertilization and cleavage rates in couples with a history of fertilization failure in ICSI treatment [3, 37]. Montag et al. distributed the cases with a history of low or failed fertilization, depending on previous fertilization rates following ICSI, and analyzed the benefit of calcium ionophore [38]. The results showed a higher fertilization rate after ICSI and AOA with calcium ionophore compared to the rate following standard ICSI in the patients with a history of <30% fertilization rate after ICSI treatment (0% versus 41.6% in patients with 0% fertilization rate after previous ICSI and 19.3% versus 44.4% in patients with 1%–29% after ICSI, respectively). Our previous research demonstrated that one long-lasting [Ca2+]i increase without repetitive spikes was recognized (Fig. 2.4b) [35].

2.3.2.3 Electrical Activation

In 1999 Yanagida et al. reported electrical oocyte activation first as piezoelectric ICSI [24]. The mechanism of oocyte activation by electrical pulse is to produce micropores in the cell membrane of oocytes to induce Ca^{2+} influx and activate the eggs. Baltaci et al. reported efficacy of piezoelectric stimulation on fertilization failure using BTX Electro Cell Manipulator with single pulse of 1.5 kV/cm DC for 100 μs in 20 min after ICSI procedure [39]. In patients with a history of fertilization failure, fertilization rate following ICSI in combination of electrical stimulation is 62% and significantly higher than that after ICSI only (62% versus 12%, respectively, $p < 0.001$). In our previous experiments, human oocytes were stimulated using an electro-cell fusion generator with single pulse of 1.2 kV/cm DC for 99 μs [40]. Figure 2.4d and e showed intracellular Ca^{2+} responses in human oocytes after electrical stimulation. Some eggs showed [Ca^{2+}]i spikes two to three times; however they were different from Ca^{2+} oscillations after ICSI.

2.3.2.4 PLCZ1 mRNA Injection

In a clinical application, we injected a candidate sperm factor, hPLCZ1 RNA (100 ng/μl), into oocytes and measured fluorescent intensity by conventional fluorescence microscopy (Fig. 2.4f). The first [Ca^{2+}]i spike occurred 23.6 min after hPLCZ1 RNA injection. After the [Ca^{2+}]i rise, repetitive transient spikes were observed. The pattern of Ca^{2+} oscillations obtained by using hPLCZ1 RNA was similar to that of Ca^{2+} oscillations in the eggs after ICSI treatment [35].

2.4 Conclusions

As shown in Table 2.1, the main cause of fertilization failure in ICSI was shown to be egg activation failure, indicating involvement of sperm factors. Oocyte activation failure can be treated by methods that directly increase [Ca^{2+}]i, such as the use of calcium ionophore. However, such AOA procedures and agents cannot form the pattern of physiological [Ca^{2+}]i increases observed at fertilization and can have potential cytotoxic or mutagenic adverse effect on eggs and embryos [3]. In contrast, the PLCZ1 RNA injection can induce optimal pattern of Ca^{2+} oscillations as that at fertilization, leading to the parthenogenetic development of blastocysts in mice, pigs, cows, monkeys, and humans [16, 41–43]. Although hPLCZ1 RNA has the ability to generate ideal and physiological egg activation, the adverse effect of RNA injection on human oocytes is still unclear. The average of RNA's half-lives is approximately 9 h [44]. Therefore, injected hPLCZ1 RNA could not exist in the ooplasm for a long time and integrate into the host genome [45–47]. Thus, injection of hPLCZ1 RNA is a potential clinical application of egg-activating agent in the future. Further studies of the safety of PLCZ1 RNA injection for human oocyte and babies are urgently needed.

References

1. Masui Y. From oocyte maturation to the in vitro cell cycle: the history of discoveries of Maturation-Promoting Factor (MPF) and Cytostatic Factor (CSF). Differentiation. 2001;69:1–17.
2. Rankin TL, Coleman JS, Epifano O, Hoodbhoy T, Turner SG, Castle PE, et al. Fertility and taxon-specific sperm binding persist after replacement of mouse sperm receptors with human homologs. Dev Cell. 2003;5:33–43.
3. Nasr-Esfahani MH, Deemeh MR, Tavalaee M. Artificial oocyte activation and intracytoplasmic sperm injection. Fertil Steril. 2010;94:520–6.
4. van der Westerlaken L, Helmerhorst F, Dieben S, Naaktgeboren N. Intracytoplasmic sperm injection as a treatment for unexplained total fertilization failure or low fertilization after conventional in vitro fertilization. Fertil Steril. 2005;83:612–7.
5. Li LJ, Zhang FB, Liu SY, Tian YH, Le F, Wang LY, et al. Human sperm devoid of germinal angiotensin-converting enzyme is responsible for total fertilization failure and lower fertilization rates by conventional in vitro fertilization. Biol Reprod. 2014;90:125.
6. Tomás C, Orava M, Tuomivaara L, Martikainene H. Low pregnancy rate is achieved in patients treated with intracytoplasmic sperm injection due to previous low or failed fertilization in invitro fertilization. Hum Reprod. 1998;13:65–70.
7. Kimura Y, Yanagimachi R. Intracytoplasmic sperm injection in the mouse. Biol Reprod. 1995;52:709–20.
8. Sasagawa I, Kuretake S, Eppig JJ, Yanagimachi R. Mouse primary spermatocytes can complete two meiotic divisions within the oocyte cytoplasm. Biol Reprod. 1998;58:248–54.
9. Mangoli V, Dandekar S, Desai S, Mangoli R. The outcome of ART in males with impaired spermatogenesis. J Hum Reprod Sci. 2008;1:73–6.
10. Yanagida K, Morozumi K, Katayose H, Hayashi S, Sato A. Successful pregnancy after ICSI with strontium oocyte activation in low rates of fertilization. Reprod Biomed Online. 2006;13(6):801.
11. Miyazaki S, Shirakawa H, Nakada K, Honda Y. Essential role fo the inositol 1,4,5-trisphosphate receptor/Ca2+ release channel in Ca2+ waves and Ca2+ oscillation of mammalian eggs. Dev Biol. 1993;158:62–78.
12. Miyazaki S, Ito M. Calcium signals for egg activation in mammals. J Pharmacol Sci. 2006;100:545–52.
13. Stricker SA. Comparative biology of calcium signaling during fertilization and egg activation in animals. Dev Biol. 1999;211:157–76.
14. Shirakawa H, Kikuchi T, Ito M. Calcium signaling in mammalian eggs at fertilization. Curr Top Med Chem. 2016;16:2664–76.
15. Swann K, Ozil JP. Dynamics of the calcium signal that triggers mammalian egg activation. Int Rev Cytol. 1994;152:183–222.

16. Saunders CM, Larman MG, Parrington J, Cox LJ, Royse J, Blayney LM, et al. PLC zeta: a sperm-specific trigger of Ca(2+) oscillations in eggs and embryo development. Development. 2002;129:3533–44.

17. Nomikos M, Kashir J, Swann K, Lai FA. Sperm PLCzeta: from structure to Ca2+ oscillations, egg activation and therapeutic potential. FEBS Lett. 2013;587:3609–16.

18. Swann K, Saunders CM, Rogers NT, Lai FA. PLCzeta(zeta): a sperm protein that triggers Ca2+ oscillations and egg activation in mammals. Semin Cell Dev Biol. 2006;17:264–73.

19. Cox LJ, Larman MG, Saunders CM, Hashimoto K, Swann K, Lai FA. Sperm phospholipase Czeta from humans and cynomolgus monkeys triggers Ca2+ oscillations, activation and development of mouse oocytes. Reproduction. 2002;124:611–23.

20. Kouchi Z, Fukami K, Shikano T, Oda S, Nakamura Y, Takenawa T, et al. Recombinant phospholipase Czeta has high Ca2+ sensitivity and induces Ca2+ oscillations in mouse eggs. J Biol Chem. 2004;279:10408–12.

21. Sanusi R, Yu Y, Nomikos M, Lai FA, Swann K. Rescue of failed oocyte activation after ICSI in a mouse model of male factor infertility by recombinant phospholipase Czeta. Mol Hum Reprod. 2015;21:783–91.

22. Knott JG, Kurokawa M, Fissore RA, Schultz RM, Williams CJ. Transgenic RNA interference reveals role for mouse sperm phospholipase Czeta in triggering Ca2+ oscillations during fertilization. Biol Reprod. 2005;72:992–6.

23. Tesarik J, Mendoza C. Spermatid injection into human oocytes. I. Laboratory techniques and special features of zygote development. Hum Reprod. 1996;11:772–9.

24. Yanagida K, Katayose H, Yazawa H, Kimura Y, Konnai K, Sato A. The usefulness of a piezo-micromanipulator in intracytoplasmic sperm injection in humans. Hum Reprod. 1999;14:448–53.

25. Kishikawa H, Wakayama T, Yanagimachi R. Comparison of oocyte-activating agents for mouse cloning. Cloning. 1999;1:153–9.

26. Murase Y, Araki Y, Mizuno S, Kawaguchi C, Naito M, Yoshizawa M, et al. Pregnancy following chemical activation of oocytes in a couple with repeated failure of fertilization using ICSI: case report. Hum Reprod. 2004;19:1604–7.

27. Szollosi MS, Kubiak JZ, Debey P, de Pennart H, Szollosi D, Maro B. Inhibition of protein kinases by 6-dimethylaminopurine accelerates the transition to interphase in activated mouse oocytes. J Cell Sci. 1993;104:861–72.

28. Cuthbertson KS, Cobbold PH. Phorbol ester and sperm activate mouse oocytes by inducing sustained oscillations in cell Ca2+. Nature. 1985;316:541–2.

29. Fissore RA, Pinto-Correia C, Robl JM. Inositol trisphosphate-induced calcium release in the generation of calcium oscillations in bovine eggs. Biol Reprod. 1995;53:766–74.

30. Steinhardt RA, Epel D. Activation of sea-urchin eggs by a calcium ionophore. Proc Natl Acad Sci U S A. 1974;71:1915–9.

31. Kuroda K, Ito M, Shikano T, Awaji T, Yoda A, Takeuchi H, et al. The role of X/Y linker region and N-terminal EF-hand domain in nuclear translocation and Ca2+ oscillation-inducing activities of phospholipase Czeta, a mammalian egg-activating factor. J Biol Chem. 2006;281:27794–805.

32. Yoon SY, Jellerette T, Salicioni AM, Lee HC, Yoo MS, Coward K, et al. Human sperm devoid of PLC, zeta 1 fail to induce Ca(2+) release and are unable to initiate the first step of embryo development. J Clin Invest. 2008;118:3671–81.

33. Heytens E, Parrington J, Coward K, Young C, Lambrecht S, Yoon SY, et al. Reduced amounts and abnormal forms of phospholipase C zeta (PLCzeta) in spermatozoa from infertile men. Hum Reprod. 2009;24:2417–28.

34. Kashir J, Jones C, Lee HC, Rietdorf K, Nikiforaki D, Durrans C, et al. Loss of activity mutations in phospholipase C zeta (PLCzeta) abolishes calcium oscillatory ability of human recombinant protein in mouse oocytes. Hum Reprod. 2011;26:3372–87.

35. Yamaguchi T, Ito M, Kuroda K, Takeda S, Tanaka A. The establishment of appropriate methods for egg-activation by human PLCZ1 RNA injection into human oocyte. Cell Calcium. 2017;65:22–30.

36. Ebner T, Moser M, Sommergruber M, Jesacher K, Tews G. Complete oocyte activation failure after ICSI can be overcome by a modified injection technique. Hum Reprod. 2004;19:1837–41.
37. Sfontouris IA, Nastri CO, Lima ML, Tahmasbpourmarzouni E, Raine-Fenning N, Martins WP. Artificial oocyte activation to improve reproductive outcomes in women with previous fertilization failure: a systematic review and meta-analysis of RCTs. Hum Reprod. 2015;30:1831–41.
38. Montag M, Koster M, van der Ven K, Bohlen U, van der Ven H. The benefit of artificial oocyte activation is dependent on the fertilization rate in a previous treatment cycle. Reprod Biomed Online. 2012;24:521–6.
39. Baltaci V, Ayvaz OU, Unsal E, Aktas Y, Baltaci A, Turhan F, et al. The effectiveness of intracytoplasmic sperm injection combined with piezoelectric stimulation in infertile couples with total fertilization failure. Fertil Steril. 2010;94:900–4.
40. Tanaka A, Nagayoshi M, Takemoto Y, Tanaka I, Kusunoki H, Watanabe S, et al. Fourteen babies born after round spermatid injection into human oocytes. Proc Natl Acad Sci U S A. 2015;112:14629–34.
41. Yoneda A, Kashima M, Yoshida S, Terada K, Nakagawa S, Sakamoto A, et al. Molecular cloning, testicular postnatal expression, and oocyte-activating potential of porcine phospholipase Czeta. Reproduction. 2006;132:393–401.
42. Rogers NT, Hobson E, Pickering S, Lai FA, Braude P, Swann K. Phospholipase Czeta causes Ca2+ oscillations and parthenogenetic activation of human oocytes. Reproduction. 2004;128:697–702.
43. Ross PJ, Beyhan Z, Iager AE, Yoon SY, Malcuit C, Schellander K, et al. Parthenogenetic activation of bovine oocytes using bovine and murine phospholipase C zeta. BMC Dev Biol. 2008;8:16.
44. Schwanhausser B, Busse D, Li N, Dittmar G, Schuchhardt J, Wolf J, et al. Global quantification of mammalian gene expression control. Nature. 2011;473:337–42.
45. Warren L, Manos PD, Ahfeldt T, Loh YH, Li H, Lau F, et al. Highly efficient reprogramming to pluripotency and directed differentiation of human cells with synthetic modified mRNA. Cell Stem Cell. 2010;7(5):618–30.
46. Goh PA, Caxaria S, Casper C, Rosales C, Warner TT, Coffey PJ, et al. A systematic evaluation of integration free reprogramming methods for deriving clinically relevant patient specific induced pluripotent stem (iPS) cells. PLoS One. 2013;8:e81622.
47. Augustyniak J, Zychowicz M, Podobinska M, Barta T, Buzanska L. Reprogramming of somatic cells: possible methods to derive safe, clinical-grade human induced pluripotent stem cells. Acta Neurobiol Exp (Wars). 2014;74:373–82.

Chapter 3
Tubal Function Abnormalities with Tubal Patency in Unexplained Infertility

Yuko Ikemoto, Keiji Kuroda, Yasushi Kuribayashi, and Masato Inoue

Abstract The fallopian tubes, or oviducts, are anatomically and functionally significant organs for successful pregnancy. They play crucial roles in the transportation of gametes and embryos and are also the sites of sperm capacitation, fertilization, and embryo development. Hysterosalpingography evaluates tubal patency but not tubal function. In unexplained infertility, a probable tubal cause of infertility is tubal function abnormality including an oocyte capture disorder in the fimbriae at ovulation and the failure to transport gametes and embryos. Treatment strategies for infertility patients with tubal dysfunction include (1) endoscopic surgery, including laparoscopy and salpingoscopy, (2) superovulation with gonadotropins and intrauterine insemination, and (3) in vitro fertilization (IVF). In younger patients with unexplained infertility who desire spontaneous pregnancy, endoscopic surgery is among the primary choices in the diagnosis of intratubal and peritubal conditions and treatment for tubal dysfunction. If patients wish to avoid endoscopic surgery or cannot conceive after such surgery, IVF is the ultimate infertility treatment. Patients with unexplained infertility who have diminished ovarian reserve or are of late reproductive age should undergo IVF as the first-line treatment.

Keywords Unexplained infertility · Fallopian tube · Oviduct · Laparoscopy Salpingoscopy · In vitro fertilization

Y. Ikemoto
Department of Obstetrics and Gynaecology, Faculty of Medicine, Juntendo University, Tokyo, Japan

K. Kuroda (✉)
Center for Reproductive Medicine and Implantation Research, Sugiyama Clinic Shinjuku, Tokyo, Japan

Department of Obstetrics and Gynaecology, Faculty of Medicine, Juntendo University, Tokyo, Japan
e-mail: arthur@juntendo.ac.jp

Y. Kuribayashi · M. Inoue
Center for Reproductive Medicine and Endoscopy, Sugiyama Clinic Marunouchi, Tokyo, Japan

© Springer Nature Singapore Pte Ltd. 2018
K. Kuroda et al. (eds.), *Treatment Strategy for Unexplained Infertility and Recurrent Miscarriage*, https://doi.org/10.1007/978-981-10-8690-8_3

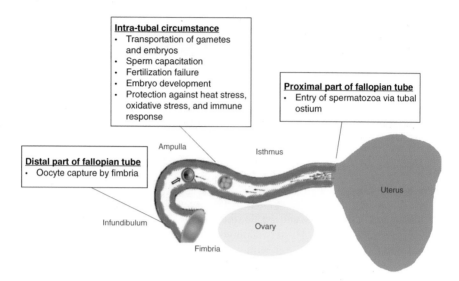

Fig. 3.1 Tubal function for pregnancy. For successful pregnancy, the fallopian tubes, or oviducts, have roles in oocyte retrieval by the fimbriae at ovulation and the transportation of gametes and are also the sites of sperm capacitation, fertilization, and embryo development

The fallopian tubes, or oviducts, are anatomically and functionally significant organs for successful pregnancy. They have roles in oocyte retrieval by the fimbriae at ovulation and the transportation of gametes and are also the sites of sperm capacitation, fertilization, and embryo development (Fig. 3.1). Hysterosalpingography (HSG) is an examination that evaluates tubal patency and anatomical abnormalities but not tubal function. Unexplained infertility can occur when a tubal function abnormality accompanies tubal patency. The candidate causes of tubal dysfunction are mainly (1) gamete and embryo transportation failure and (2) tubal fimbria dysfunction in oocyte retrieval. Herein, we review tubal function and disorders in unexplained infertility.

3.1 Oviduct Anatomy and Disorders

The oviducts are reproductive organs with abundant blood flow that connect the uterus and the ovaries. Each oviduct consists, distally to proximally, of fimbriae, an infundibulum, an ampulla, and an isthmus and has four histological layers including, from outer to inner, the serosa, muscle, submucosa, and mucosa. Compared with those in the ampulla and fimbriae, the smooth muscles in the tubal isthmus are well developed. Secretory cells in the oviduct produce oviduct fluid, which plays a role in gamete and embryo transportation via ciliary movement. Compared with the

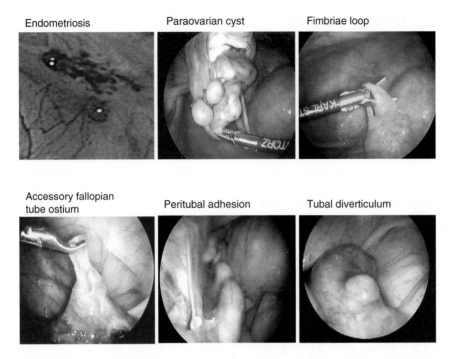

Fig. 3.2 Tubal anatomical variations. The figure shows images of tubal or pelvic anatomical variations including peritoneal lesions of endometriosis, accessory fallopian tube ostium, paraovarian cyst, peritubal adhesions, fimbriae loop, and tubal diverticulum

isthmus, the tubal ampulla has abundant ciliated cells. The proper number, structure, and orientation of the cilia are critical for oviduct transport functions [1].

HSG and laparoscopic chromotubation testing can evaluate tubal patency. However, HSG has reported sensitivity of 65% and specificity of 83% for tubal patency and peritubal adhesions [2]. Thus, the precise detection of tubal patency with HSG is difficult, yet the high specificity of this approach makes it an efficient test for diagnosing tubal occlusion despite the lower reliability for detecting peritubal adhesion. Two reports evaluating the use of HSG in the laparoscopic assessment of infertile women with tubal patency showed a high frequency of abnormal intrapelvic findings such as endometriosis (31–64%) and peritubal adhesion or tubal occlusion (14–16%) [3, 4].

Infertile women often have tubal or pelvic anatomical variations including accessory fallopian tube ostium, paraovarian cyst, peritubal adhesions, and tubal diverticulum (Fig. 3.2) [5–8]. However, it remains unclear whether these abnormalities cause infertility; therefore, laparoscopic surgery to restore fallopian tube function may be an appropriate treatment for oocyte retrieval disorder, thereby leading to successful pregnancy in women with unexplained infertility.

3.2 Oviduct Function and Disorders

3.2.1 Transportation of Gametes and Embryos

At ovulation, oocytes are captured by the tubal fimbriae and transported toward the ampulla via oviduct fluid flow. Oviduct fluid is generated from secretory cells and flows via ciliary movement and the contraction of tubal muscles. On the contrary, when ejaculated sperm enter the tubal isthmus via the tubal ostium, sperm hyperactivation is induced through interaction with epithelial cells in the oviduct. The activated sperm move with rotation against the oviduct fluid toward the ampulla for fertilization [9, 10]. The thermosensing capability of the sperm allows them to reach the ampulla along an oviduct temperature gradient [11].

Embryos are transported through the oviduct toward the uterus by myosalpinx contractions, ciliary movement, and oviduct fluid flow [1, 12]. Estradiol (E_2) contributes to embryo transportation, whereas progesterone (P4) has the opposite effect. E_2 and P4 orchestrate embryo transportation toward the uterus by regulating the contraction of tubal muscles, movement of ciliated epithelial cells, and secretion and flow of oviduct fluid [1, 13, 14].

3.2.2 Protection Against Heat Stress, Oxidative Stress, and Maternal Immune Response

The oviduct also protects gametes and embryos from heat stress, oxidative stress, and maternal immune rejection. Oviductal epithelial cells produce heat shock proteins to reduce heat stress, and oviduct fluid contains proteins that defend against oxidative stress, such as albumin, transferrin, catalase, and superoxide dismutase. The concentration of oviduct fluid protein is the lowest at ovulation and highest at the time of menstruation [15]. The oviducts can sense the resultant change in viscosity during the menstrual cycle and adjust the flow rate by increasing ciliary movement [16]. The fallopian tube can also sense the existence of sperm and control the protein and antioxidant concentrations in the oviduct fluid, possibly to support for reduction of sperm stress [17]. Moreover, the oviducts protect embryos against own immunological rejection through E_2 signaling [1, 18–21].

3.2.3 Capacitation

Capacitation is the maturation process of sperm, which is required for the acrosome reaction and acquisition of the capability to penetrate an oocyte. Compared with unattached sperm, human sperm attached to the oviductal epithelium has a greater incidence of hyperactivation in the capacitation process. Oviduct epithelial cells and their cross talk with embryos are also keys for capacitation [22, 23].

3.2.4   Embryo Development

Oviduct fluid is associated with embryo development. During the earliest stages, embryos remain in the oviduct for 3–4 days [24]. Various components for regulating embryo development, including growth factors, transferrin, and albumin as embryotropic factors, have been identified in oviduct fluid [1]. Cleavage-stage embryos require pyruvate, lactate, and glycogen, and during the morula and blastocyst stages, the mitochondria in embryos are matured and changed by glycolytic metabolism. The co-culture of early mouse and human embryos and tubal epithelial cells significantly increases the rates of embryo cleavage and blastocyst development, which suggests that oviductal epithelial cells are important for embryonic development [25].

3.3   Candidate Causes of Tubal Dysfunction in Unexplained Infertility

3.3.1   Oocyte Capture Dysfunction in Tubal Fimbriae

The tubal function of oocyte capture can be impaired by anatomical adhesions caused by endometriosis or *Chlamydia trachomatis* infection. Various inflammatory cytokines and macrophages in the intrapelvic fluid of women with endometriosis prevent the fimbrial cilia from attaching to the cumulus oophorus, which inhibits oocyte capture [26]. Internal pressure in the tubal ampulla is also required for oocyte capture [27], and minor tubal abnormalities (see Fig. 3.2) may be associated with aberrant tubal pressure.

3.3.2   Transportation Failure of Gametes or Embryos

Embryos and gametes are transported through the oviduct via oviduct fluid flow, temperature gradients, chemical attractants, ovarian steroids, myosalpinx contractions, and ciliary movement [12]. Out of unexplained infertility, tubal transportation failure, but not occlusion, may result from abnormalities of the interior of the fallopian tube, such as the loss or rounded edges of tubal mucosal folds and the presence of adhesions, abnormal vessels, or debris (Fig. 3.3). Salpingitis is one cause of abnormalities of the oviduct interior. A wide variety of microorganisms, such as *Escherichia coli*, *Staphylococcus aureus*, *Neisseria gonorrhea*, *C. trachomatis*, and *Mycobacterium tuberculosis*, can cause salpingitis. *E. coli* or *S. aureus* infections cause acute salpingitis with prominent clinical manifestations such as lower abdominal pain and fever during the early period of infection. However, salpingitis caused by *N. gonorrhea*, *C. trachomatis*, or *M. tuberculosis* lacks obvious symptoms and

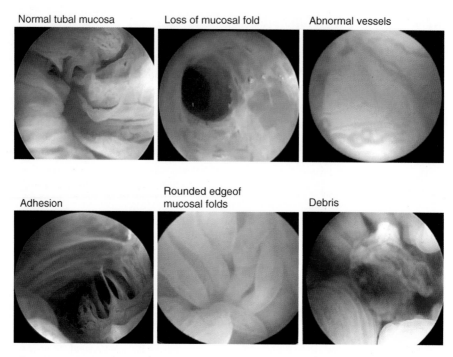

Fig. 3.3 Salpingoscopic findings in the tubal lumen. The figure demonstrates images of intratubal findings using salpingoscopy. Abnormalities of the interior of the fallopian tube include the loss or rounded edges of tubal mucosal folds and the presence of adhesions, abnormal vessels, or debris

often shifts asymptomatically to chronic salpingitis. *C. trachomatis* infection induces the loss of epithelial cell microvilli and cilia that is reversible with early and appropriate antibiotic treatment [28]. However, once the shift to chronic salpingitis occurs, inflammation spreads to the subcutaneous stroma of the oviducts and induces irreversible functional disorders and oviductal stenosis. Moreover, after the remission of acute salpingitis, chronic salpingitis may continue due to the autoimmunity acquired through infection with *C. trachomatis*. The immune response to heat shock protein 60 by *C. trachomatis* is related to a delayed-type hypersensitivity reaction and may promote damage to oviductal epithelial cells [29].

3.3.3 Endometriosis

Endometriosis has detrimental effects on the oviducts that hamper their functions in sperm motility and embryonic development owing to the development of intrapelvic adhesions and chronic inflammation with inflammatory cytokines and macrophages [30]. Compared with patients without endometrioma, infertility patients with ovarian endometrioma have a lower prevalence of intratubal findings such as loss of mucosal folds (24.1% and 46.8%, respectively, $p < 0.05$), which suggests that infertile patients with endometriosis are likely to have normal oviducts [31]. Therefore, in patients with endometriosis, infertility or subfertility may arise owing to intrapelvic inflammation, not tubal dysfunction. Intact fallopian tubes may also induce the development of endometriosis through retrograde menstrual bleeding.

3.3.4 Smoking

Smoking is a risk factor for tubal pregnancy and infertility [32] through a mechanism that remains poorly understood. A complex mixture of toxic chemicals is found in tobacco smoke. Furthermore, nicotine influences tubal motility, structure, and blood flow as well as oocyte capture by the fimbriae [33–35]. A recent study showed that cigarette smoking decreases tubal motility and changes the tubal microenvironment via the reduced expression of the pro-apoptotic gene *BAD* and the induction of survival-related gene *BCL2* expression [33]. However, no changes in the ciliated cells of the fallopian tubes in women with smoking have been identified [36].

3.4 Treatment Strategies

3.4.1 Endoscopic Surgery

Laparoscopic surgery for patients with unexplained infertility may contribute to successful pregnancy outcomes if mild endometriosis or peritubal adhesion is identified and treated. Shimizu et al. compared pregnancy outcomes in unexplained infertility women after laparoscopic surgery followed by infertility treatment (laparoscopy group) and infertility treatment alone (nonlaparoscopy group; Fig. 3.4) [37]. In the laparoscopy group, endometriosis was found in 62.7% of patients, adhesions of the adnexa were found in 7.8%, and both lesions were found in 11.8%. After laparoscopy, 31.4% of women conceived spontaneously. However, after in vitro fertilization (IVF), cumulative pregnancy rates in both groups reached 60% at 1-year posttreatment. Therefore, in younger patients with unexplained infertility who desire spontaneous pregnancy, laparoscopic surgery is one of the primary treatment options [37].

Franjoine et al. demonstrated the efficacy of laparoscopic fimbrioplasty for the treatment of unexplained infertility in patients aged ≤35 years. Fimbrioplasty dilates and expands the surface area of the tubal fimbriae by gently opening the fimbrial lumens several times using a right-angle cystic duct clamp. At 1 year of follow-up, patients with unexplained infertility who underwent laparoscopic fimbrioplasty had a cumulative pregnancy rate without IVF that was significantly higher than that in the group that underwent diagnostic laparoscopy alone (51.5% versus 28.8%, respectively, $p = 0.02$). The rates in both groups plateaued at

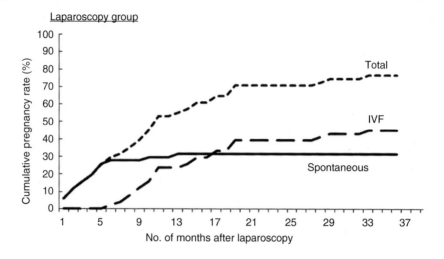

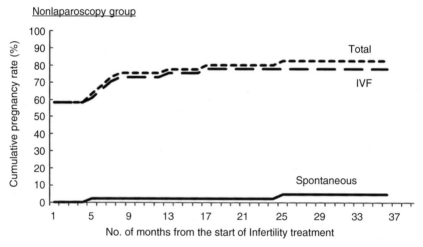

Fig. 3.4 Cumulative pregnancy rate after laparoscopic surgery in unexplained infertility patients. A study by Shimizu et al. examined pregnancy outcomes in women with unexplained infertility after laparoscopic surgery followed by infertility treatment (laparoscopy group) and infertility treatment alone (nonlaparoscopy group). After laparoscopy, 31.4% of the subjects conceived spontaneously. However, when the patients in both groups underwent in vitro fertilization, the groups reached a cumulative pregnancy rate of >60% in 1 year

6–7 months. However, no significant difference in outcomes was observed for patients aged >35 years. Women aged ≤35 years in the surgery group had an overall pregnancy rate (per cycle) that was significantly higher than that in the control group (22.7% versus 13.3%, respectively, $p = 0.06$; Fig. 3.5) [38].

Salpingoscopy or falloposcopy can evaluate various intratubal findings such as adhesions, mucosal fold changes, and debris (see Fig. 3.2), and salpingoscopic surgery mainly comprises fallopian tube recanalization using balloon catheters for

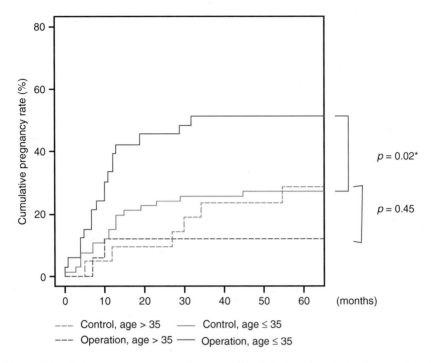

Fig. 3.5 Cumulative pregnancy rate after laparoscopic fimbrioplasty in patients with unexplained infertility or mild endometriosis. In a study by Franjoine et al., patients aged ≤35 years with unexplained infertility that was significantly higher who underwent laparoscopic fimbrioplasty (51.5%) had a cumulative pregnancy rate without assisted reproductive technology higher that was than that of the control group (diagnostic laparoscopy alone) at 1 year after treatment (51.5% versus 28.8%, respectively, $p = 0.02$). The rates in both groups plateaued in 6–7 months. No significant difference in rates was observed in women aged >35 years

proximal tubal obstruction or stenosis. Dechaud et al. investigated the difference in spontaneous pregnancy rates in patients with unexplained infertility diagnosed by HSG or laparoscopy and "true" unexplained infertility without intratubal findings on falloposcopy (Fig. 3.6). In the unexplained infertility patients without intratubal abnormalities elucidated by falloposcopic findings, the spontaneous pregnancies occur at a higher rates of 28.6% and 33.3% during the first 4 months and 24 months of follow-up, respectively, after the procedure, comparing to those of unexplained infertility diagnosed by HSG or laparoscopy (see Fig. 3.6) [39].

3.4.2   Superovulation with Gonadotropins and Intrauterine Insemination

In patients with unexplained infertility, the cumulative pregnancy rate after timed intercourse or intrauterine insemination (IUI) or mild ovarian stimulation is 10–20%,

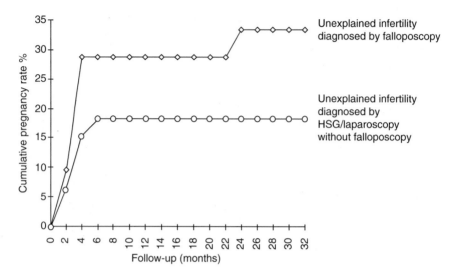

Fig. 3.6 Cumulative spontaneous pregnancy rates in patients with unexplained infertility diagnosed by hysterosalpingography (HSG) or laparoscopy and "true" unexplained infertility without intratubal findings on falloposcopy. In the unexplained infertility patients without intratubal abnormalities, the spontaneous pregnancies occur at a higher rates of 28.6% and 33.3% during the first 4 months and 24 months of follow-up, respectively, after the procedure, comparing to those of unexplained infertility diagnosed by HSG or laparoscopy

which is comparable with that of expectant management [40, 41]. However, the combination treatment of superovulation with gonadotropins and IUI produces cumulative pregnancy rates of 50–60% [40, 41]. A large number of injected spermatozoa and ovulated eggs may overcome mild oviduct dysfunction or endometriosis. The incidence of ovarian hyperstimulation syndrome is low, but multiple pregnancies occur at a high rate of 6–35% after these treatments [40, 41]. Therefore, patients should be informed about the risk of multiple conceptions before undergoing ovarian stimulation.

3.4.3 In Vitro Fertilization

If patients with unexplained infertility wish to avoid endoscopic surgery or cannot conceive after such surgery, IVF is the ultimate treatment. The National Institute for Health and Clinical Excellence guidelines also recommend IVF if the duration of infertility is ≥2 years [42]. Hughes et al. reported that the likelihood of live birth during the first cycle of IVF was 20.9-fold higher than that in subfertile couples with tubal patency in a randomized controlled trial [43]. A review by Tsafrir et al. showed that IVF is the first-line treatment for women with unexplained infertility who are aged >40 years owing to the low efficacy and poor pregnancy outcomes of ovulation induction and IUI, which advance ovarian aging [44].

3.5 Conclusion

Evaluations of the oviducts and peritubal environment with laparoscopy and salpingoscopy are keys for patients with unexplained infertility who desire spontaneous pregnancy. Furthermore, endoscopic surgery can benefit certain infertile patients with minor tubal abnormalities and mild endometriosis. Patients with diminished ovarian reserves and those of late reproductive age should proceed directly to IVF.

References

1. Li S, Winuthayanon W. Oviduct: roles in fertilization and early embryo development. J Endocrinol. 2017;232:R1–R26.
2. Swart P, Mol BW, van der Veen F, van Beurden M, Redekop WK, Bossuyt PM. The accuracy of hysterosalpingography in the diagnosis of tubal pathology: a meta-analysis. Fertil Steril. 1995;64:486–91.
3. Tsuji I, Ami K, Miyazaki A, Hujinami N, Hoshiai H. Benefit of diagnostic laparoscopy for patients with unexplained infertility and normal hysterosalpingography findings. Tohoku J Exp Med. 2009;219:39–42.
4. Bélisle S, Collins JA, Burrows EA, Willan AR. The value of laparoscopy among infertile women with tubal patency. J SOGC. 1996;18:326–36.
5. Yablonsk M, Sarge T, Wild RA. Subtle variations in tubal anatomy in infertile women. Fertil Steril. 1990;54:455–8.
6. Cohen BM, Katz M. The significance of the convoluted oviduct in the infertile woman. J Reprod Med. 1978;21:31–5.
7. Beyth Y, Kopolovic J. Accessory tubes: a possible contributing factor in infertility. Fertil Steril. 1982;38:382–3.
8. Siddhartha C, Rajib GC, Sandip D, Vishnu P. Minor tubal defects—the unnoticed causes of unexplained infertility. J Obstet Gynaecol India. 2010;60:331–6.
9. Morales P, palma V, Salgado M, Villalón M. Fertilization and early embryology: sperm interaction with human oviductal cells in vitro. Hum Reprod. 1996;11:1504–9.
10. Miki K, Clapham DE. Rheotaxis guides mammalian sperm. Curr Biol. 2013;23:443–52.
11. Bahat A, Caplan SR, Eisenbach M. Thermotaxis of human sperm cells in extraordinarily shallow temperature gradients over a wide range. PLoS One. 2012;7:e41915.
12. Ezzati M, Djahanbakhch O, Arian S, Carr BR. Tubal transport of gametes and embryos: a review of physiology and pathophysiology. J Assist Reprod Genet. 2014;31:1337–47.
13. Orihuela PA, Ríos M, Croxatto HB. Disparate effects of estradiol on egg transport and oviductal protein synthesis in mated and cyclic rats1. Biol Reprod. 2001;65:1232–7.
14. Cretoiu SM, Cretoiu D, Suciu L, Popescu LM. Interstitial Cajal-like cells of human Fallopian tube express estrogen and progesterone receptors. J Mol Histol. 2009;40:387–94.
15. Lippes J, Krasner J, Alfonso LA, Dacalos ED, Lucero R. Human oviductal fluid proteins. Fertil Steril. 1981;36:623–9.
16. Andrade YN, Fernandes J, Vázquez E, Fernández-Fernández JM, Arniges M, Sánchez TM, Villalón M, Valverde MA. TRPV4 channel is involved in the coupling of fluid viscosity changes to epithelial ciliary activity. J Cell Biol. 2005;168:869–74.
17. Georgiou AS, Sostaric E, Wong CH, Snijders AP, Wright PC, Moore HD, Fazeli A. Gametes alter the oviductal secretory proteome. Mol Cell Proteomics. 2005;4:1785–96.
18. Mariani ML, Ciocca DR, Gonzalez Jatuff AS, Souto M. Effect of neonatal chronic stress on expression of Hsp70 and oestrogen receptor alpha in the rat oviduct during development and the oestrous cycle. Reprodoction. 2003;126:801–8.

19. Guérin P, El Mouatassim S, Ménézo Y. Oxidative stress and protection against reactive oxygen species in the pre-implantation embryo and its surroundings. Hum Reprod Update. 2001;7:175–89.
20. Wira CR, Fahey JV, Sentman CL, Pioli PA, Shen L. Innate and adaptive immunity in female genital tract: cellular responses and interactions. Immunol Rev. 2005;206:306–35.
21. Winuthayanon W, Bernhardt ML, Padilla-Banks E, Myers PH, Edin ML, Lih FB, Hewitt SC, Korach KS, Williams CJ. Oviductal estrogen receptor alpha signaling prevents protease-mediated embryo death. Elife. 2015;4:e10453.
22. Suarez SS. Control of hyperactivation in sperm. Hum Reprod Update. 2008;14:647–57.
23. Kervancioglu ME, Djahanbakhch O, Aitken RJ. Epithelial cell coculture and the induction of sperm capacitation. Fertil Steril. 1994;61:1103–8.
24. Croxatto HB. Physiology of gamete and embryo transport through the fallopian tube. Reprod Biomed Online. 2002;4:160–9.
25. Takeuchi K, Nagata Y, Sandow BA, Hodgen GD. Primary culture of human fallopian tube epithelial cells and co-culture of early mouse pre-embryos. Mol Reprod Dev. 1992;32:236–42.
26. Suginami H, Yano K. An ovum capture inhibitor (OCI) in endometriosis peritoneal fluid: an OCI-related membrane responsible for fimbrial failure of ovum capture**supported in part by the grant-in-aid for scientific research no. 62570761 from the Japanese Ministry of Education, Science and Culture. Fertil Steril. 1988;50:648–53.
27. Osada H, Fujii TK, Tsunoda I, Takagi K, Satoh K, Kanayama K, Endo T. Fimbrial capture of the ovum and tubal transport of the ovum in the rabbit, with emphasis on the effects of beta 2-adrenoreceptor stimulant and prostaglandin F2 alpha on the intraluminal pressures of the tubal ampullae. J Assist Reprod Genet. 1999;16:373–9.
28. Cooper MD, Rapp J, Jeffery-Wiseman C, Barnes RC, Stephens DS. Chlamydia trachomatis infection of human fallopian tube organ cultures. J Gen Microbiol. 1990;136:1109–15.
29. Lichtenwalner AB, Patton DL, Van Voorhis WC, Sweeney YT, Kuo CC. Heat shock protein 60 is the major antigen which stimulates delayed-type hypersensitivity reaction in the macaque model of Chlamydia trachomatis salpingitis. Infect Immun. 2004;72:1159–61.
30. Harada T, Iwabe T, Terakawa N. Role of cytokines in endometriosis. Fertil Steril. 2001;76:1–10.
31. Nakagawa K, Nishi Y, Sugiyama R, Kuribayashi Y, Akira S, Sugiyama R, Inoue M. Role of salpingoscopy in assessing the inner fallopian tubes of infertility patients with ovarian endometriomas. J Obstet Gynaecol Res. 2013;39:979–84.
32. Farquhar CM. Ectopic pregnancy. Lancet. 2005;366:583–91.
33. Horne AW, Brown JK, Nio-Kobayashi J, Abidin HB, Adin ZE, Boswell L, Burgess S, Lee KF, Duncan WC. The association between smoking and ectopic pregnancy: why nicotine is BAD for your fallopian tube. PLoS One. 2014;9:e89400.
34. Mitchell JA, Hammer RE. Effects of nicotine on oviducal blood flow and embryo development in the rat. J Reprod Fertil. 1985;74:71–6.
35. Knoll M, Talbot P. Cigarette smoke inhibits oocyte cumulus complex pick-up by the oviduct in vitro independent of ciliary beat frequency. Reprod Toxicol. 1998;12:57–68.
36. Pier B, Kazanjian A, Gillette L, Strenge K, Burney RO. Effect of cigarette smoking on human oviductal ciliation and ciliogenesis. Fertil Steril. 2013;99:199–205.
37. Shimizu Y, Yamaguchi W, Takashima A, Kaku S, Kita N, Murakami T. Long-term cumulative pregnancy rate in women with unexplained infertility after laparoscopic surgery followed by in vitro fertilization or in vitro fertilization alone. J Obstet Gynaecol Res. 2011;37(5):412.
38. Franjoine SE, Bedaiwy MA, AbdelHafez FF, Geng C, Liu JH. Clinical effectiveness of modified laparoscopic fimbrioplasty for the treatment of minimal endometriosis and unexplained infertility. Minim Invasive Surg. 2015;2015:730513.
39. Dechaud H, Daures JP, Hedon B. Prospective evaluation of falloposcopy. Hum Reprod. 1998;13:1815–8.
40. Gunn DD, Bates GW. Evidence-based approach to unexplained infertility: a systematic review. Fertil Steril. 2016;105:1566–74.e1.

41. Chaffkin LM, Nulsen JC, Luciano AA, Metzger DA. A comparative analysis of the cycle fecundity rates associated with combined human menopausal gonadotropin (hMG) and intra-uterine insemination (IUI) versus either hMG or IUI alone. Fertil Steril. 1991;55:252–7.
42. NICE. National Institute for Health and Clinical Excellence. National Collaborating Centre for Women's and Children's Health. Fertility: assessment and treatment for people with fertility problems. 2013;156:63.
43. Hughes EG, Beecroft ML, Wilkie V, Burville L, Claman P, Tummon I, Greenblatt E, Fluker M, Thorpe K. A multicentre randomized controlled trial of expectant management versus IVF in women with Fallopian tube patency. Hum Reprod. 2004;19:1105–9.
44. Tsafrir A, Simon A, Margalioth EJ, Laufer N. What should be the first-line treatment4for unexplained infertility in women over 40 years of age - ovulation induction and IUI, or IVF? Reprod Biomed Online. 2009;19(Suppl 4):4334.

Chapter 4
Implantation Failure 1: Intrauterine Circumstances and Embryo–Endometrium Synchrony at Implantation

Keiji Kuroda and Satoko Yamashita

Abstract The causes of recurrent implantation failure (RIF) include chronic endometritis, cesarean scar syndrome, and embryo–endometrial asynchrony at implantation such as impaired decidualization of the uterine endometrium. The gold standard treatments for chronic endometritis and cesarean scar syndrome are broad-spectrum antibiotics and hysteroscopic surgery, respectively. The optimal window of implantation (WOI) can be identified with an endometrial receptivity array or nucleolar channel system test. If optimal WOI is detected, the best strategy for patients with a history of RIF is frozen-warmed single-blastocyst transfer.

Keywords Recurrent implantation failure · Chronic endometritis · Cesarean scar syndrome · Endometrial receptivity array · In vitro fertilization · Window of implantation

In recent years, the quality and frequency of in vitro fertilization (IVF) have rapidly grown; however, overcoming recurrent implantation failure (RIF) and multiple IVF failures with high-quality or chromosomally normal embryos is difficult with common IVF procedures. The causes of RIF include uterine inhibitory factors of implantation without embryo origin. Here we introduce three maternal causes of implantation failure: chronic endometritis (CE), cesarean scar syndrome, and

K. Kuroda (✉)
Center for Reproductive Medicine and Implantation Research, Sugiyama Clinic Shinjuku, Tokyo, Japan

Department of Obstetrics and Gynaecology, Faculty of Medicine, Juntendo University, Tokyo, Japan
e-mail: arthur@juntendo.ac.jp

S. Yamashita
Department of Obstetrics and Gynecology, Faculty of Medicine, Oita University, Yufu-shi, Oita, Japan

Department of Obstetrics and Gynaecology, Faculty of Medicine, Juntendo University, Tokyo, Japan

© Springer Nature Singapore Pte Ltd. 2018   33
K. Kuroda et al. (eds.), *Treatment Strategy for Unexplained Infertility and Recurrent Miscarriage*, https://doi.org/10.1007/978-981-10-8690-8_4

embryo–endometrial asynchrony at implantation, including impaired decidualization of the uterine endometrium.

4.1 Chronic Endometritis

A persistent inflammation of the local endometrium, CE occurs in approximately 30–60% of women with a history of RIF [1–4]. CE that is asymptomatic and undetectable with general fertility tests is characterized by the presence of plasma cells in biopsied endometrial samples [5]. A wide variety of microorganisms, such as *Escherichia coli*, *Enterococcus faecalis*, *Gardnerella vaginalis*, *Streptococcus* spp., *Mycoplasma* spp., and *Chlamydia trachomatis*, are responsible for CE [3]. Some biopsied endometrial samples from patients with CE contain plasmacytes alone, and no bacteria are detected [1, 3]; therefore, the gold standard for CE diagnosis is histopathological verification via immunostaining with the plasmacyte marker CD138 [5]. Hysteroscopy is also a reliable tool for CE diagnosis [6, 7]. Typical hysteroscopic findings are an erythrogenic endometrial surface with multiple white spots, known as "strawberry aspect," and micropolyps (Fig. 4.1) [8]. The diagnostic accuracy of hysteroscopy is >90% when important findings such as hyperemia, stromal edema, and micropolyps are present [7].

Erythrogenic surface   Stromal edema

Mycropolyps

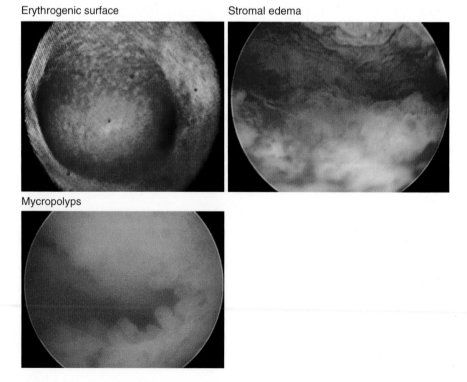

Fig. 4.1 Hysteroscopic finding of chronic endometritis. Typical hysteroscopic findings are an erythrogenic endometrial surface with multiple white spots, known as "strawberry aspect" (left panel), stromal edema (right panel) and micropolyps (lower panel)

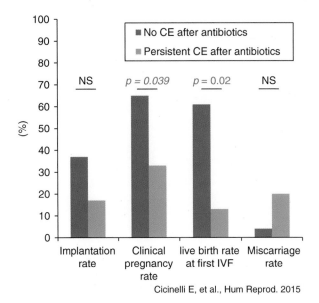

Cicinelli E, et al., Hum Reprod. 2015

Fig. 4.2 Outcomes of the first in vitro fertilization cycle after the treatment for chronic endometritis (CE). The number of previous in vitro fertilization attempts and number of transferred embryos were 4.1 times and 1.9 embryos, respectively, in both groups. In patients with recurrent implantation failure (RIF), clinical pregnancy and live birth rates are significantly higher in patients without CE compared with those with persistent CE. The miscarriage rate is relatively lower in women with RIF who do not have CE. Cicinelli et al., Hum Reprod. 2015

The recommended treatment for CE is broad-spectrum antibiotics against a wide range of bacteria. Oral doxycycline, 100 mg twice a day for 2 weeks, is the first choice, and a combination of ciprofloxacin (500 mg) and metronidazole (500 mg) twice a day for 2 weeks is the second choice [1]. Kitaya et al. investigated the overall cure rates of CE in patients with a history of RIF following antibiotic therapy and reported rates of 92.3% and 99.1% after the first-line doxycycline treatment and the second-line combined ciprofloxacin/metronidazole treatment, respectively [9]. This antibiotic treatment protocol offers a high likelihood of recovery from CE, which leads to improvements in clinical pregnancy rates. Cicinelli et al. compared the outcomes of initial IVF treatments in patients with RIF and without persistent CE and those with CE who underwent antibiotic therapy (Fig. 4.2). The clinical pregnancy and live birth rates per embryo transfer (ET) were significantly higher in patients without CE than in those with persistent CE [10]. Regarding IVF treatment cycles in patients with RIF, the optimal diagnosis and treatment of CE can dramatically improve the live birth rate.

In women with endometriosis, menstrual blood and eutopic endometrium contain high levels of various bacteria [11, 12]. Thus patients with RIF and endometriosis should be examined for CE. The transplantation hypothesis posits that endometriosis occurs via retrograde menstruation and is the most widely accepted explanation for the condition. The establishment of an ectopic endometrium as endometriosis may develop from shed inflammatory endometrium that contains bacteria. However, intrauterine operations for examinations of CE such as endometrial biopsy and

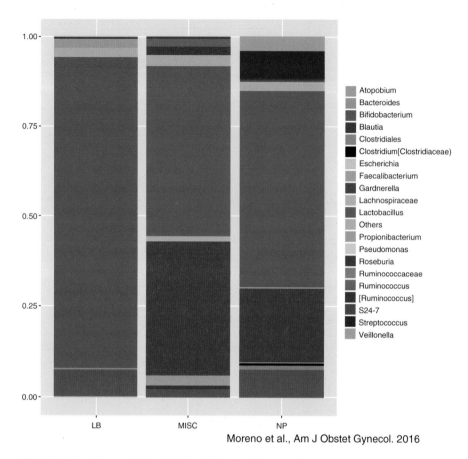

Moreno et al., Am J Obstet Gynecol. 2016

Fig. 4.3 Microbiome analysis of endometrial microbiota. Analysis of the endometrial microbiota in fertile women revealed *Lactobacillus*-enriched microbial communities. Microbiome analysis of endometrial biopsies from patients with a history of miscarriage or implantation failure showed a low abundance of endometrial *Lactobacillus*. Patients are categorized into three groups according to the reproductive outcome: *LB* live birth, *MISC* biochemical pregnancy or clinical miscarriage, and *NP* nonpregnant. Moreno et al., Am J Obstet Gynecol. 2016

hysteroscopy are risk factors for the development of tubo-ovarian abscesses in patients with ovarian endometrioma [13]. Therefore, we recommend examining the intrauterine endometrium with utmost caution after preventive antibiotic treatment.

Recent studies have described a new technology, microbiome analysis, that can sequence the 16S ribosomal RNA in each bacterium present at a sampling site. Analysis of the endometrial microbiota in fertile women demonstrated that *Lactobacillus*-enriched microbial communities (≥90%) are characteristic and related to endometrial receptivity [14]. In patients with a history of miscarriage in a previous pregnancy or implantation failure after ET, the microbiome analysis of endometrial biopsies showed that the microbiota contained a large proportion of *Gardnerella* and *Streptococcus* and that the composition of their microbiota was significantly different from that of fertile women (Fig. 4.3) [14]. Microbiome analysis may become a clinical tool for determining the individual character of endometrial microbiota.

4.2 Cesarean Scar Syndrome

A higher incidence of secondary infertility is observed in patients with a history of cesarean section than in those who deliver vaginally [15]. Secondary infertility in women with abnormal postmenstrual uterine bleeding and a prior delivery by cesarean section can be caused by bloody fluid from a cesarean scar defect (CSD) that prohibits implantation. The trapped blood in CSD may flow into the vagina as genital spotting and the intrauterine cavity, affecting the character of the cervical mucus, sperm transport, and implantation [16]. This mechanism of implantation failure is similar to that caused by hydrosalpinx. The scar dimple is known by various names such as CSD, isthmocele, sacculation, and uterine diverticulum [17].

Morris was the first to give the name "cesarean scar syndrome" to the disorder derived from cesarean scar [18, 19]. The prevalence of CSD is 24–84% in women with a history of one or more deliveries by cesarean section [17]. Furthermore, 29–82% of women with CSDs have postmenstrual uterine spotting [17]. The risk factors associated with cesarean scar syndrome include multiple cesarean deliveries, retroversion of the uterus, and use of surgical techniques such as single-layer closure during cesarean section [20]. Most patients with cesarean scar syndrome labored before cesarean section [21]. When cesarean section is performed during cervical dilation by labor, the incision may be closer to the internal uterine ostium than it is during a scheduled delivery, which in turn leads to CSD development.

Transvaginal ultrasound, saline infusion sonohysterography, or magnetic resonance imaging can identify CSDs (Fig. 4.4). The timing of the attempts for detecting CSDs is crucial, because bloody fluid is trapped in the scar between menstruation and ovulation but not during the luteal phase. Hysteroscopy also provides significant data for the direct confirmation of CSDs. The scar is generally erythrogenic with dendritic vessels (see Fig. 4.4).

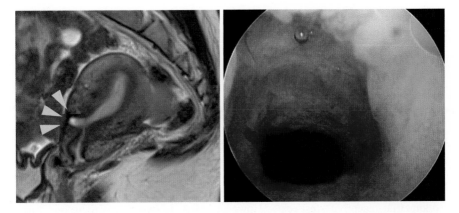

Fig. 4.4 Examination findings in cesarean scar syndrome. Magnetic resonance imaging shows a cesarean scar defect (left panel, yellow arrows). Hysteroscopy shows an erythrogenic scar (right panel)

Fig. 4.5 Hysteroscopic surgery for cesarean scar syndrome. The purpose of hysteroscopic surgery for cesarean scar syndrome is resecting the inferior and superior edges of the scar defect (*dotted line*) and cauterizing the neovascularity

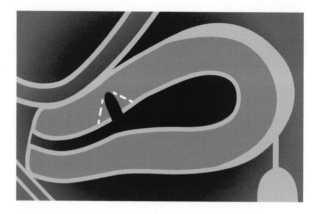

The current standard treatment for cesarean scar syndrome is hysteroscopic surgery for resecting the inferior and superior edges of CSD and cauterizing its neovascularity (Fig. 4.5). Gubbini et al. performed a prospective study of hysteroscopic surgery and reported a 100% clinical pregnancy rate within 24 months after the operation (90.2% delivery and 9.8% spontaneous abortion in 41 patients) [16]. If residual myometrial CSD is extremely thin, the scar should be resected and sutured laparoscopically. Tanimura et al. reported that the procedure was limited to patients with 2.5-mm residual myometrial thicknesses [22]. When the thickness was <2.5 mm, CSD was resected and sutured using a combination of laparoscopy and hysteroscopy. Notably, if the uterus was retroverted, the bilateral round ligaments of the uterus were shortened with sutures and anteflexed to prevent CSD recurrence. In 63.6% of patients (14 of 22 cases), successful pregnancy occurred within 1 year. No patients delivered with uterine rupture after undergoing this surgical procedure.

4.3 Embryo–Endometrial Asynchrony (Impaired Decidualization of the Endometrium)

Embryonic implantation requires mutual interaction and synchronization between a morphologically and developmentally competent embryo and an optimally decidualized endometrium. Noyes defined the dynamic and complex changes in the human endometrium during the menstrual cycle as endometrial dating [23, 24]. The window of implantation (WOI), which is the period of receptivity for blastocyst implantation, occurs through the decidual transformation of endometrium. WOI can be subjectively identified through endometrial dating of immunostained endometrial tissues. Endometrial receptivity array (ERA) is a tool for objectively identifying optimal WOI based on 238 genes identified from a microarray analysis of decidualizing human endometrium (Fig. 4.6) [25, 26]. This novel test is offered by IGENOMIX and is available in the public domain (http://www.igenomix.com/tests/endometrial-receptivity-test-era/). However, ERA is expensive; therefore, cost-effectiveness must be considered before its utilization.

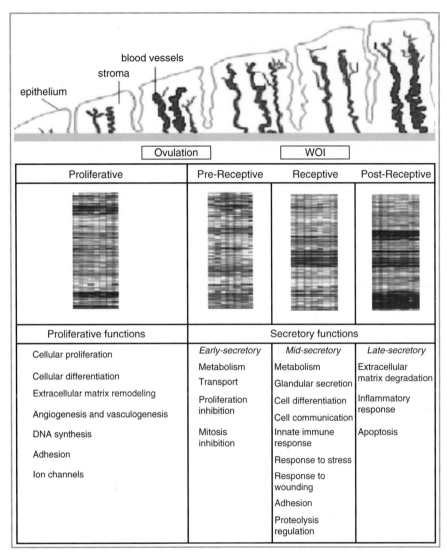

Garrido-Gómez, et al., Fertil Steril. 2013

Fig. 4.6 Gene profiles of an endometrial receptivity array (ERA) during menstruation. A heat map shows ERA gene expression profiles during the menstrual cycle and the biological functions at each stage of menstruation (proliferative, pre-receptive, receptive, and post-receptive)

The nucleolar channel system (NCS) comprises membranous organelles of epithelial cell nuclei that briefly appear during WOI (Fig. 4.7) [27, 28]. Nejat et al. confirmed the concordance between ERA results and the results of immunofluorescence staining of NCS during WOI [29]. The identification of NCS is as effective as ERA for detecting the optimal WOI. Thus, the immunofluorescence staining of NCS may also become a future clinical tool for confirming individual WOIs.

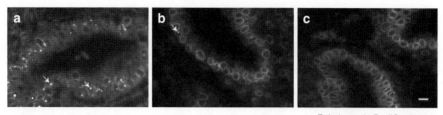

Rybak, et al., FertilSteril. 2011

Fig. 4.7 Immunofluorescence staining of the nucleolar channel system (NCS). Representative images of NCS showing "receptive" (left panel), low (center panel), and "nonreceptive" (right panel) endometrium. Rybak et al., Fertil Steril. 2011

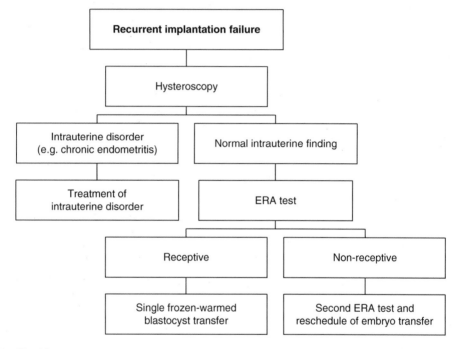

Fig. 4.8 Treatment strategy for recurrent implantation failure in women with suspected embryo–endometrial asynchrony. After hysteroscopy, the optimal window of implantation (WOI) is identified using an endometrial receptivity array (ERA) or nucleolar channel system (NCS) test. If the result is "nonreceptive," the optimal WOI must be validated with a second test. When the result is "receptive," the best strategy is frozen-warmed embryo transfer using a single high-quality (or chromosomally normal) blastocyst

The treatment strategy for RIF related to suspected embryo–endometrial asynchrony is shown in Fig. 4.8. Intrauterine conditions are first confirmed with hysteroscopy. CE is one of the causes of impaired endometrial decidualization [30]. When intrauterine finding is normal, an ERA or NCS confirmation can be used to determine whether the decidualized endometrium is optimal for implantation. If ERA or

NCS testing indicates that the endometrium is "nonreceptive," the optimal WOI must be validated with a second test, and the timing of ET must be rescheduled.

When the endometrium is "receptive," we recommend the transfer of a single frozen-warmed blastocyst. Controlled ovarian stimulation for multiple follicle development adversely affects endometrial receptivity owing to the influence of supraphysiologic levels of abnormal endocrine hormones on the proliferative and decidualizing processes of the endometrium [31–33]. A recent meta-analysis showed that frozen-warmed embryos result in higher implantation rates [34, 35]. When a pregnancy test is negative after the transfer of a cleaved embryo, determining whether cleavage arrest or impaired endometrial receptivity is responsible for implantation failure is impossible. Therefore, embryos used for treating RIF should be cultured until the blastocyst stage. The results of some studies have suggested that poor-quality embryos have adverse effects on implantation [36, 37]. Thus, the implantation rate after double ET with low- and high-quality embryos is lower than that after elective single ET [38]. ET with multiple embryos is also not recommended. The best treatment strategy for patients with a history of RIF is frozen-warmed ET of one high-quality (or chromosomally normal) blastocyst into a receptive endometrium.

References

1. Johnston-MacAnanny EB, Hartnett J, Engmann LL, Nulsen JC, Sanders MM, Benadiva CA. Chronic endometritis is a frequent finding in women with recurrent implantation failure after in vitro fertilization. Fertil Steril. 2010;93:437–41.
2. Kitaya K, Tada Y, Taguchi S, Funabiki M, Hayashi T, Nakamura Y. Local mononuclear cell infiltrates in infertile patients with endometrial macropolyps versus micropolyps. Hum Reprod. 2012;27:3474–80.
3. Kitaya K, Matsubayashi H, Yamaguchi K, Nishiyama R, Takaya Y, Ishikawa T, Yasuo T, Yamada H. Chronic endometritis: potential cause of infertility and obstetric and neonatal complications. Am J Reprod Immunol. 2016;75:13–22.
4. Kushnir VA, Solouki S, Sarig-Meth T, Vega MG, Albertini DF, Darmon SK, Deligdisch L, Barad DH, Gleicher N. Systemic inflammation and autoimmunity in women with chronic endometritis. Am J Reprod Immunol. 2016;75:672–7.
5. McQueen DB, Perfetto CO, Hazard FK, Lathi RB. Pregnancy outcomes in women with chronic endometritis and recurrent pregnancy loss. Fertil Steril. 2015;104:927–31.
6. Cicinelli E, De Ziegler D, Nicoletti R, Colafiglio G, Saliani N, Resta L, Rizzi D, De Vito D. Chronic endometritis: correlation among hysteroscopic, histologic, and bacteriologic findings in a prospective trial with 2190 consecutive office hysteroscopies. Fertil Steril. 2008;89:677–84.
7. Cicinelli E, Resta L, Nicoletti R, Tartagni M, Marinaccio M, Bulletti C, Colafiglio G. Detection of chronic endometritis at fluid hysteroscopy. J Minim Invasive Gynecol. 2005;12:514–8.
8. Bouet PE, El Hachem H, Monceau E, Gariepy G, Kadoch IJ, Sylvestre C. Chronic endometritis in women with recurrent pregnancy loss and recurrent implantation failure: prevalence and role of office hysteroscopy and immunohistochemistry in diagnosis. Fertil Steril. 2016;105:106–10.
9. Kitaya K, Matsubayashi H, Takaya Y, Nishiyama R, Yamaguchi K, Takeuchi T, Ishikawa T. Live birth rate following oral antibiotic treatment for chronic endometritis in infertile

women with repeated implantation failure. Am J Reprod Immunol. 2017;78(5). https://doi. org/10.1111/aji.12719.

10. Cicinelli E, Matteo M, Tinelli R, Lepera A, Alfonso R, Indraccolo U, Marrocchella S, Greco P, Resta L. Prevalence of chronic endometritis in repeated unexplained implantation failure and the IVF success rate after antibiotic therapy. Hum Reprod. 2015;30:323–30.

11. Khan KN, Kitajima M, Hiraki K, Yamaguchi N, Katamine S, Matsuyama T, Nakashima M, Fujishita A, Ishimaru T, Masuzaki H. Escherichia coli contamination of menstrual blood and effect of bacterial endotoxin on endometriosis. Fertil Steril 2010;94:2860–3.e1–3.

12. Khan KN, Fujishita A, Kitajima M, Hiraki K, Nakashima M, Masuzaki H. Intra-uterine microbial colonization and occurrence of endometritis in women with endometriosisdagger. Hum Reprod. 2014;29:2446–56.

13. Terao M, Koga K, Fujimoto A, Wada-Hiraike O, Osuga Y, Yano T, Kozuma S. Factors that predict poor clinical course among patients hospitalized with pelvic inflammatory disease. J Obstet Gynaecol Res. 2014;40:495–500.

14. Moreno I, Codoner FM, Vilella F, Valbuena D, Martinez-Blanch JF, Jimenez-Almazan J, Alonso R, Alama P, Remohi J, Pellicer A, Ramon D, Simon C. Evidence that the endometrial microbiota has an effect on implantation success or failure. Am J Obstet Gynecol. 2016;215:684–703.

15. LaSala AP, Berkeley AS. Primary cesarean section and subsequent fertility. Am J Obstet Gynecol. 1987;157:379–83.

16. Gubbini G, Centini G, Nascetti D, Marra E, Moncini I, Bruni L, Petraglia F, Florio P. Surgical hysteroscopic treatment of cesarean-induced isthmocele in restoring fertility: prospective study. J Minim Invasive Gynecol. 2011;18:234–7.

17. Tulandi T, Cohen A. Emerging manifestations of cesarean scar defect in reproductive-aged women. J Minim Invasive Gynecol. 2016;23:893–902.

18. Morris H. Surgical pathology of the lower uterine segment caesarean section scar: is the scar a source of clinical symptoms? Int J Gynecol Pathol. 1995;14:16–20.

19. Morris H. Caesarean scar syndrome. S Afr Med J. 1996;86:1558.

20. Tower AM, Frishman GN. Cesarean scar defects: an underrecognized cause of abnormal uterine bleeding and other gynecologic complications. J Minim Invasive Gynecol. 2013;20:562–72.

21. Armstrong V, Hansen WF, Van Voorhis BJ, Syrop CH. Detection of cesarean scars by transvaginal ultrasound. Obstet Gynecol. 2003;101:61–5.

22. Tanimura S, Funamoto H, Hosono T, Shitano Y, Nakashima M, Ametani Y, Nakano T. New diagnostic criteria and operative strategy for cesarean scar syndrome: endoscopic repair for secondary infertility caused by cesarean scar defect. J Obstet Gynaecol Res. 2015;41:1363–9.

23. Noyes RW, Haman JO. Accuracy of endometrial dating; correlation of endometrial dating with basal body temperature and menses. Fertil Steril. 1953;4:504–17.

24. Noyes RW, Hertig AT, Rock J. Dating the endometrial biopsy. Am J Obstet Gynecol. 1975;122:262–3.

25. Diaz-Gimeno P, Horcajadas JA, Martinez-Conejero JA, Esteban FJ, Alama P, Pellicer A, Simon C. A genomic diagnostic tool for human endometrial receptivity based on the transcriptomic signature. Fertil Steril. 2011;95:50–60.

26. Garrido-Gomez T, Ruiz-Alonso M, Blesa D, Diaz-Gimeno P, Vilella F, Simon C. Profiling the gene signature of endometrial receptivity: clinical results. Fertil Steril. 2013;99:1078–85.

27. Guffanti E, Kittur N, Brodt ZN, Polotsky AJ, Kuokkanen SM, Heller DS, Young SL, Santoro N, Meier UT. Nuclear pore complex proteins mark the implantation window in human endometrium. J Cell Sci. 2008;121:2037–45.

28. Rybak EA, Szmyga MJ, Zapantis G, Rausch M, Beshay VE, Polotsky AJ, Coutifaris C, Carr BR, Santoro N, Meier UT. The nucleolar channel system reliably marks the midluteal endometrium regardless of fertility status: a fresh look at an old organelle. Fertil Steril. 2011;95:1385–9.e1.

29. Nejat EJ, Ruiz-Alonso M, Simon C, Meier UT. Timing the window of implantation by nucleolar channel system prevalence matches the accuracy of the endometrial receptivity array. Fertil Steril. 2014;102:1477–81.
30. Wu D, Kimura F, Zheng L, Ishida M, Niwa Y, Hirata K, Takebayashi A, Takashima A, Takahashi K, Kushima R, Zhang G, Murakami T. Chronic endometritis modifies decidualization in human endometrial stromal cells. Reprod Biol Endocrinol. 2017;15:16.
31. Roque M, Lattes K, Serra S, Sola I, Geber S, Carreras R, Checa MA. Fresh embryo transfer versus frozen embryo transfer in in vitro fertilization cycles: a systematic review and meta-analysis. Fertil Steril. 2013;99:156–62.
32. Horcajadas JA, Pellicer A, Simon C. Wide genomic analysis of human endometrial receptivity: new times, new opportunities. Hum Reprod Update. 2007;13:77–86.
33. Kolibianakis E, Bourgain C, Albano C, Osmanagaoglu K, Smitz J, Van Steirteghem A, Devroey P. Effect of ovarian stimulation with recombinant follicle-stimulating hormone, gonadotropin releasing hormone antagonists, and human chorionic gonadotropin on endometrial maturation on the day of oocyte pick-up. Fertil Steril. 2002;78:1025–9.
34. Dieamant FC, Petersen CG, Mauri AL, Comar V, Mattila M, Vagnini LD, Renzi A, Petersen B, Nicoletti A, Oliveira JBA, Baruffi RL, Franco JG Jr. Fresh embryos versus freeze-all embryos – transfer strategies: nuances of a meta-analysis. JBRA Assist Reprod. 2017;21:260–72.
35. Coates A, Kung A, Mounts E, Hesla J, Bankowski B, Barbieri E, Ata B, Cohen J, Munne S. Optimal euploid embryo transfer strategy, fresh versus frozen, after preimplantation genetic screening with next generation sequencing: a randomized controlled trial. Fertil Steril. 2017;107:723–30.e3.
36. Brosens JJ, Salker MS, Teklenburg G, Nautiyal J, Salter S, Lucas ES, Steel JH, Christian M, Chan Y-W, Boomsma CM, Moore JD, Hartshorne GM, Sucurovic S, Mulac-Jericevic B, Heijnen CJ, Quenby S, Koerkamp MJG, Holstege FCP, Shmygol A, Macklon NS. Uterine selection of human embryos at implantation. Sci Rep. 2014;4:3894.
37. Teklenburg G, Salker M, Molokhia M, Lavery S, Trew G, Aojanepong T, Mardon HJ, Lokugamage AU, Rai R, Landles C, Roelen BAJ, Quenby S, Kuijk EW, Kavelaars A, Heijnen CJ, Regan L, Brosens JJ, Macklon NS. Natural selection of human embryos: decidualizing endometrial stromal cells serve as sensors of embryo quality upon implantation. PLoS One. 2010;5:e10258.
38. Wintner EM, Hershko-Klement A, Tzadikevitch K, Ghetler Y, Gonen O, Wintner O, Shulman A, Wiser A. Does the transfer of a poor quality embryo together with a good quality embryo affect the In Vitro Fertilization (IVF) outcome? J Ovarian Res. 2017;10:2.

Chapter 5
Implantation Failure 2: Immunomodulating Treatment for the Patients with Repeated Implantation Failures Caused by Immunological Rejection

Koji Nakagawa and Rikikazu Sugiyama

Abstract Although the repeated implantation failures (RIF) in assisted reproductive technology field could cause many different reasons, the reaction that women could immunologically reject the embryos has been well known to be one of the reasons of RIF. Recently, it is reported that the balance of T-helper 1 (Th1) and T-helper 2 (Th2) has a potential to become a useful marker for detecting immunological rejection between the uterine endometrium of the infertile women and transferred embryos in ART treatment. Moreover, this ratio can be used for choosing the treatment strategy for the patients for RIF. The immunological rejection as a cause of RIF is not majority, but this cause can be solved by the appropriate approach. In this chapter, the immunomodulation treatment from the old fashion such as glucocorticoid and intravenous immunoglobulin G to the current one such as TNF-α and tacrolimus is introduced and shown how to use them. In particular, tacrolimus treatment is very useful and effective for the patients with RIF and also unexplained recurrent pregnancy loss and is safe for both mothers and fetus. The methods of using tacrolimus for the patients with RIF and RPL are interpreted in detail.

Keywords Immunological rejection · IVIG · Glucocorticoid · Immunological rejection · Immunomodulation therapy · Tacrolimus · TNF-α inhibitor

5.1 Introduction

Depending on definition used, about 10% of couples who received in vitro fertilization (IVF) treatment will experience recurrent implantation failures (RIF), and many of them who can achieve implantation will be disappointed in early pregnancy

K. Nakagawa (✉) · R. Sugiyama
Center for Reproductive Medicine and Implantation Research, Sugiyama Clinic Shinjuku, Tokyo, Japan
e-mail: koji@sugiyama.or.jp

© Springer Nature Singapore Pte Ltd. 2018
K. Kuroda et al. (eds.), *Treatment Strategy for Unexplained Infertility and Recurrent Miscarriage*, https://doi.org/10.1007/978-981-10-8690-8_5

45

loss [1]. The patients who failed to get pregnancy even though receiving a lot of high-quality embryos want to know the reasons why they have failed. When the clinicians faced these RIF patients, they try to search for something to improve the success, and they sometimes might choose the several strategies for these patients without confident theoretical explanation. These strategies include several immuno-modulation treatments; however, those are selected as not theoretical but empirical treatments.

To modulate immune response between maternal endometrium and the implant-ing embryo makes the clinicians rouse their interest in this field. The first step for this process is to understand how the mother immunologically tolerates a geneti-cally alien embryo and what has happened at the spot of invasion of maternal tissues by the embryo. One of the mechanisms, which help for understanding the ideas about a balance between pro- and anti-inflammatory states, is characterized by a palette of cytokines and immune cells such as T-helper cells and natural killer (NK) cells, which can influence the fate of the implanting embryo. While it is becoming clear the function of these cytokines, the repeated failures of IVF can gradually be solved by the concepts about immune reaction such as immune rejection and immune tolerance between the uterine endometrium and implanting or implanted embryos.

In this chapter, the immunomodulation treatments which are currently performed in the IVF fields for the patients with RIF or recurrent miscarriages (RM) in the IVF fields are introduced. The many studies trying to prove the efficacy of various immunomodulation therapies, which are heterogeneous in design, method, inter-vention, and study population, make it difficult to explain and understand them. We need a profound understanding on both mechanisms and modulations about human implantation when we are trying to make progress in this field. Therefore, immuno-modulation treatments fascinate the doctors who face the patients with RIF. We make sure that this chapter shows a brief summary for the current use of immuno-modulation treatments supported by the published evidence and will be helpful for both the patients who are suffering from RIF and the clinicians who face these patients.

5.2 The Theoretical Mechanisms for Using Immunomodulation Drug

The success of implantation is realized that hatched blastocyst can reach the surface of the endometrium and invade in the decidualized endometrium. During the blasto-cyst development, the vascularization and remodeling of the spinal arteries occurred; consequently the maternal-fetal circulation is established. Immune cells act as key worker in the maternal response to the blastocyst, and a lot of studies have focused the importance of a balanced cytokine environment. Currently, the balance between T-helper 1 (Th1) and T-helper 2 (Th2) produced cytokines as determinations of implantation become popular. The Th1 and Th2 cell ratio is a useful marker to evaluate either stronger rejection or reduced tolerance. A shift in the ratio toward Th1 cells leads to increased production of pro-inflammatory cytokines such as tumor necrosis factor alpha (TNF-α), interferon gamma (INF-γ), and interleukin (IL)-2, which play important parts of cytotoxic immune response, phagocytosis, and inflammation. On the other hand, Th2 cells produce a variety of interleukins acting as the humoral immune response and inhibit several functions of phagocytosis, which are one of anti-inflammatory responses [2]. These theoretical mechanisms demonstrated a number of observational studies reporting increased expression of pro-inflammatory cytokines in women with a history of recurrent pregnancy loss [3].

The uterine NK (uNK) cells have elevated during the implantation and early pregnancy period. After ovulation, uNK cells increase as the dominant immune cells in the uterine endometrium changed after decidualization [4]. Moreover, the uNK cells expand surrounding the trophoblast cells in the decidualized endometrium in early gestation. Therefore, it is thought that the uNK cells play an important role to control of establishment of placenta by keeping a balance between normal and excessive invasion of trophoblast to the uterine endometrium. On the other hand, peripheral blood NK cells act in the innate immune system to recognize foreign cells without showing HLA-class I molecules and early killing of viral pathogens; however, they might be not key factors of endometrial function [4], and they might stimulate antigen-presenting cells; therefore they activate adaptive immune system.

There is a different idea on the local balance between pro- and anti-inflammation induced by several cytokines in the perceptive uterine endometrium. The decrease of anti-inflammatory cytokines at the maternal-fetal face is explained as an idea, being simpleminded [5–7]. The study about cytokine concentration of the fluid from uterine cavity in 201 women before ET was performed, and authors showed a positive relationship between IL-10 and TNF-α around both implantation and early pregnancy period. In contrast, a negative relationship was observed between secretions of IL-1β and monocyte chemoattractant protein 1 levels around implantation and early pregnancy period [8].

The many reports demonstrated that the relationship between increase of peripheral blood NK cells and Th1/Th2 cell ratio [2, 9–11] among women showing RIF or with recurrent pregnancy loss (RPL) has motivated us to measure peripheral NK cell, but there is little relationship between the peripheral blood NK cells and uNK cells [4, 7]. Tuckerman and co-workers indicated that the RIF patients showed a higher count of uNK cells in their endometrium [12]. To evaluate NK cells which are taken from the peripheral blood or uterine endometrium becomes useful for searching the causes of RIF or RPL in the maternal site. These examinations make us support or help to select a better method for the patients suffering from RIF or RPL among various immunomodulation treatments or drugs. Many immunomodulation treatments are introduced, which act via immunological response such as reducing rejection or strengthening tolerance; consequently the uterine endometrium can accept the blastocyst or not reject fetus.

5.3 Glucocorticoids

Corticosteroid treatment shows a lot of features during implantation period and early pregnancy, to suppress both immune cell activity and numbers. The taking process of this corticosteroid is simple, and the cost of this treatment is cheaper than the other immunomodulation drugs, and this drug acts rapidly and might be safe; therefore this is easily prescribed. Since the use of this corticosteroid treatment is widespread, this is easily included as interventions even though the many studies which tried to prove the efficacy of aspirin or low molecular weight heparin (LMWH) for the immunomodulation treatment for the women with RIF or RPL were performed. We wonder whether the corticosteroid is effective or not. A meta-analysis of randomized controlled trials (RCTs) was reported to indicate the effect of glucocorticoid treatment for the patients who have undergone IVF of intracytoplasmic sperm injection (ICSI) [13]. In this article, the glucocorticoids were used during implantation period, and 13 studies were suitable for its analysis, in which 1759 participants were enrolled. There is no significant difference in both live-birth and pregnancy rates between the treatment and control groups [14–16]. But these reports did not mention about treatment period of glucocorticoid and infertility causes in the analysis and the participants' background such as with RIF or not. Another seven studies reported the miscarriage rate [14–19]; those showed no statistically significant difference on miscarriage rate between the treatment and control groups. There is only one study indicating that glucocorticoids can prevent ovarian hyperstimulation syndrome (OHSS) [20]. Moreover, the incidence of this complication using glucocorticoid is not increased.

On the other hand, glucocorticoid is effective for the infertility patient showing positive autoantibodies. It is easily thought that autoantibodies can affect both implanting and implanted embryos, because these embryos are semi-allograft. The glucocorticoid is one of the treatment choices for the patients with RIF or RPL [21], endometriosis, and unexplained infertility [22, 23]. Corticosteroids suppress autoantibodies, which form a small clot in the peripheral blood vessel to combine to the platelet and endothelial membrane phospholipids, and may improve pregnancy outcomes of patients experiencing RPL with autoantibodies. For RIF patients with autoantibodies [24] or patients with antinuclear antibodies [25], this treatment gave steady results. One randomized trial which examined whether glucocorticoid treatment was beneficial for the patients with positive autoantibodies or not was performed and reported that the pregnancy rate in the treatment group administrated with 5 mg daily dose of prednisolone was significantly higher than that in the control group even though autoantibody titers did not decrease [14]. Another randomized trial trying to confirm the efficacy of this treatment in patients with endometriosis was performed and showed that the pregnancy rate did not increase in the intervention group compared to the control group [18].

According to these reports, glucocorticoid treatment is identified to be effective for certain patient group such as possessing autoantibodies, but drawing the conclusions that glucocorticoid treatment can improve pregnancy outcome among the patients with RIF or RPL might be premature judgment; therefore, another randomized control trial using double blinded and placebo is needed. Summarizing the reports mentioned above about glucocorticoid treatment for the patients with RIF or RPL, no apparent evidence is seen that theoretically persuades the clinicians who empirically use glucocorticoid for the patients with RIF and RPL. Glucocorticoids, which act as an anti-inflammatory agent, are not favorable to use during the peri-implantation period, because the implantation is thought to the area of inflammation, and to suppress the inflammatory reaction might interfere implantation.

5.4 Heparin Treatment

Heparin treatment has been often used as the treatment for the RIF patients. Because of its antithrombotic effect, the expected effect is large, but this drug works as a certain immunological positive effect to induce implantation [26]. Heparin shows several positive effects on implantation as follows. One of the actions of this drug is prevention of complement activation among expectant women showing antiphospholipid antibodies [27]. Moreover, the heparin-binding epidermal growth factor can improve an invasive trophoblast and prevent apoptosis [28]. Heparin also increases the insulin-like growth factor (IGF) I and IGF II levels, those that induce irruption of trophoblast [26]. Heparin shows facilitating transcription of matrix metalloproteinases that might regulate interactions between embryo and decidualized endometrium inducing invasion of trophoblast. Besides these effects, low cost and simple administration were its characteristics.

There were several reports to evaluate the effects of heparin treatments for the patients with repeated implantation failure in ART treatment [27–31]; however, most of them showed no significant differences in ART outcomes between the treatment with heparin and control groups. Moreover, these studies did not indicate the clear criteria to start heparin treatment such as showing at least one thrombophilia disorder. And the conclusion drawn here is that a certain immunological positive effect of heparin for RIF patients is weak because glucocorticoids were used as a cotreatment among three report.

5.5 Aspirin

Acetylsalicylic acid (ASA), which is famous as aspirin, has been used as a painkilling anti-inflammatory agent for a long time, and more recently it is well known to prevent cardiovascular disease and widely used. ASA can suppress the prostaglandins' products to reduce the cyclooxygenase activity, especially in platelets. This suppression is an irreversible change and leads to inhibit the thromboxane synthesis, resulting to protect vascular constriction. The use of ASA is expected to inhibit inflammation during the implantation period or early pregnancy in the uterine endometrium, and this inhibition helps the embryo to invade into the endometrium [32, 33]. Although there are many reports to try to prove the effect of ASA for the RIF patients, the Cochrane review mentioned that the patients who received ART treatment administrated by ASA during the implantation period could not increase the pregnancy outcomes including clinical pregnancy, ongoing pregnancy, or live-birth rates [34]. But the published reports showed various protocols, subjects, dosage and duration, monitoring indices, and other concomitant drugs; therefore results from these reports were difficult to understand, even though this treatment was confirmed to bring good effects for some women's groups, who showed problems such as possessing antiphospholipid antibodies or blood coagulation disorders.

5.6   Immunoglobulin G

It is well known that the treatment using intravenous administration of immunoglobulin G (IVIG) got good results among the patients who have autoimmune antibodies or showing inflammatory status such as recurrent inflammatory polyneuropathy, Guillain-Barre syndrome, and Kawasaki disease [35]. In a reproductive field, the IVIG is expected to reduce peripheral cytotoxic NK cells [36], strengthen regulatory T cell power, and suppress B cell function [37]. From these results, it was suggested that the IVIG treatment might change immunological conditions from elevated Th1/Th2 balance by the dominance of Th1 cells to appropriate this balance reducing Th1 cell count. Therefore, this change might weaken immunological refection and raise immunological tolerance.

There were only two RCTs by a MEDLINE search, and one was performed in which IVIG was administrated to human. According to this RCT, patients who experienced ≥2 times of implantation failures administrated 500 mg/kg IVIG, on the day of ET. They could receive the same dose of IVIG after 4 weeks when they achieved pregnancy and the fetal heartbeat was confirmed. This study could not indicate that IVIG improved the ART outcomes regarding clinical pregnancy, implantation, and live-birth rates between the intervention and control groups [38].

After the previous study was published, three papers were published about the administration of IVIG for the patients with RIF [37, 39, 40]. Although these reports resulted that IVIG treatment was favorable, they had several problems that might involve the results in each report. The study published by Ramos-Medina and coworkers [37] was conducted as an observational cohort study. They retrospectively analyzed 428 patients who experienced multiple IVF failures or pregnancy losses, showing elevated NK cell count or NKT-like lymphocyte. These patients were administrated with IVIG 400 mg/kg at the timing of embryo transfer, and they received IVIG after positive pregnancy test and continuously administrated every 3 weeks until 35–36 weeks of gestation. In this study, all patients received low-dose aspirin (100 mg/day) even though they are showing no abnormal coagulation ability, and some of them showing clotting disorder received both low-dose aspirin and

Table 5.1 Characteristics of various immunomodulation treatments

	IVIG[a]	Anti-TNF-α (Adalimumab)	Intralipid	Tacrolimus
Product	Veniron®, Gurovenin®	Humira®	Intralipos injection 10%	Prograf®
Route of administration	Intravenous	Intravenous	Intravenous	Oral
Dose	400–500 mg/kg/ once	40 mg, twice, 2-week interval	10% 250 ml/ day	1–3 mg/day
Start	The day of ET	90–120 days before ET	After OPU	2 days before ET day
After positive pregnancy test	Continued, every 3–4 weeks	None	Continued, every 2 weeks	Continued
Monitor:	Peripheral NK cell count, Th1/Th2 ratio	Th1/Th2ratio	Peripheral NK cell count	Th1/Th2ratio, Th1 level
Concern	Risk of infection of human parvovirus B19, plasma fraction, hyperviscosity	Immunosuppressive interstitial pneumonia	Soybean allergy	Contraindication during pregnancy
Cost	Expensive About 2300 USD/ once	Expensive About 600 USD/ once	Cheap About 6 USD/once	Expensive 50–150 USD/ week

[a]*IVIG* intravenous immunoglobulin

heparin. The authors in this report indicated a higher pregnancy and live-birth rates in the treatment group compared to the control group with significant difference. Winger et al. try to divide the IVIG intervention group by the results of diagnostic peripheral blood examinations which might become a good marker of this IVIG treatment to predict the results. They mentioned that the administration of IVIG might be effective for one RIF subgroup showing elevated Th1/Th2 cell ratio or an increased CD56+ CD3- cell population [41, 42]. These indices might become a marker for this IVIG treatment.

A current review concluded that IVIG treatment might benefit for subgroups to improve implantation, pregnancy, and live-birth rates [43]. This IVIG treatment for the patients with RIF might be selected without selecting available treatments, because the patients have to receive some burden from this treatment, such as its cost and risk (Table 5.1). The cost of IVIG of one treatment estimates 2000 USD (i.e., patient's BW = 50 kg), and immunoglobulin is one of the blood fraction products, and it is not assured about contamination of viral infection (i.e., human parvovirus B19). The patients have to receive additional IVIG treatment after positive pregnancy test, and this treatment has to be continued until the third trimester. Since the treatment with IVIG makes the patients bear the expenses and receive intravenous infusion, we should be careful to choose this treatment, and we have to select this treatment when the benefit is thought to be bigger than the burden for the patients compared to other immunomodulation treatments.

5.7   Anti-TNF-α (Adalimumab)

Tumor necrosis factor α (TNF-α) that is one of the cytokines belonging to the TNF superfamily is produced by the macrophage and differentiates and induces Th1 cell from naive T cell. Adalimumab, which is a recombinant human TNF-α monoclonal antibody, has an effect for the patients with rheumatoid arthritis, psoriasis, and inflammatory bowel disease. This drug is effective to inhibit the function of TNF-α to combine with TNF-α receptor, consequently suppressing the inflammatory signals via Th1 cell and destroying the TNF-producing cell.

Currently, there are no randomized trials to evaluate the efficacy of this drug (anti-TNF-α antibody drug) for the patients who received ART treatment. A few reports could be found using this drug in the ART field [41–44]. Winger and co-workers conducted a cohort study, in which the patients were prospectively divided into four groups according to the combination of the administrated drugs. The authors used the two types of cytokine combination patterns, TNF-α and IL-10 or INF-γ/IL-10 to select patients; subsequently patients <38 years showing both high Th1 and Th2 cell ratio (INF-γ/IL-10 ≥ 30.6 and INF-γ/IL-10 ≥ 20.5) were selected. The patients in the group I received both TNF-α and intravenous immunoglobulin, the patients in the group II were treated with only intravenous immunoglobulin, the patients on the group III received only TNF-α, and the patients in the group IV received no treatment. The patients belonging to these groups were treated with heparin, with or without showing thrombophilia. The participants possess morphologically good embryos. The treatment groups (group I, II, and III) improve the ART outcomes regarding the implantation, clinical pregnancy, and live-birth rates compared to the group IV with no medication [41]. Another paper from the same authors was published. Patients <40 years showing high Th1/Th2 cell ratio were recruited and were administrated both with anti-TNF-α drug and LWMH, and the women without high Th1/Th2 ratio were as control. The authors evaluated the ART outcomes retrospectively, and they revealed that the patients who received anti-TNF-α drug showed better ART outcomes (higher implantation, clinical pregnancy, and live-birth rates) compared to the control group. However, this positive result is low evidence level due to its poor protocol and makes us difficult to trust their results [42].

One of the most unfavorable reactions from adalimumab is immunosuppressive reaction. Adalimumab is usually administrated by intravenous infusion, and it is impossible to adjust the given dose; therefore, the patients faced the risk of immunosuppressive reaction. Adalimumab is effective to inhibit the function of TNF-α to combine with TNF-α receptor, consequently suppressing the inflammatory signals via Th1 cell and destroying the TNF-producing cell; as a result of this reaction, immunosuppressive condition will be established. In this situation, the patients who received adalimumab might have a risk of viral and bacterial infections. The published reports showed low evidence level and have some problems in each study; therefore, we cannot give adequate information of this treatment for the patients; moreover, there is no method to select patients who are effective for this adalimumab. From these reasons, at present this adalimumab is not recommended as a treatment for the patients with RIF or RPL.

5.8 Intralipid

Intralipid, which is a 20% fat emulsion comprised of soybean oil, egg phospholipids, and glycerin, is one of the useful methods for the patients who cannot take any meal, and its immunosuppressive effect was historically revealed by an elevated rate of bacteria in neonates [45]. Intralipid was first suggested as a potential therapy for recurrent miscarriage in 1994 after a miscarriage rate of only 30% was reported in 20 control patients who received intralipid [46]. Further in vivo study in human indicated that intralipid can suppress blood natural killer cell cytotoxicity [47]. The first clinical report was published by Ndukwe and co-workers where 50 RIF patients with immune dysfunction had 50% live-birth rate with intralipid therapy [48]. There have since been two RCTs, each involving over 200 patients, which both reported statistical benefit [49, 50]. Dakhly and co-workers demonstrated a RCT to evaluate the effects of intralipid therapy for the unexplained infertility or repeated pregnancy loss of patients [50]. In this study, participants showing elevated NK cell activity were recruited and divided into two groups randomly, a treatment group which consisted of patients who received 250 ml of intralipid and the control group which included patients receiving 250 ml of saline, at the day of oocyte pickup day. After establishment of achieving pregnancy, the same infusion was performed every 2 weeks until 14 weeks of gestation. In this report, the authors could not show a higher hCG-positive rate in the treatment group compared to the control group, but about ongoing pregnancy rate in the treatment group, they could show a higher rate than that in the control group [50], but this difference was weak due to the number of participants. This intralipid infusion is safe for the patients, but there is no theological explanation for the effect of this treatment. The author did not mention the reason why the treatment group showed significantly higher ongoing and live-birth rates than those of the patients' group without treatment. Does intralipid work as an immunomodulation drug? The clinicians easily cannot use it for the patients without clarifying the mechanism of increasing implantation by intralipid.

5.9 Tacrolimus

T-helper lymphocytes are usually classified into mainly two subtypes according to their ability to produce cytokines: T-helper 1 (Th1) or T-helper 2 (Th2) cells [1, 51]. In immunological rejection or tolerance, Th1 and Th2 cells act as the leading characters

[52]. It is thought as common sense that the establishment of pregnancy is immuno-logical condition that Th2 shows superiority over Th1; in contrast the condition that Th1 shows superiority over Th2 is immunological rejection; consequently, this Th1 superiority can reject transferred embryos [1, 53]. From this theory, the implantation failures are thought to be alike the allograft rejection [54]; therefore when embryos which are transferred into the uterine endometrium could not be immunologically rejected, this reaction is considered to be similar to the allograft rejection.

Recently, the advance of the new immunosuppressive drugs can achieve higher graft survival rate in the organ transplantation [55]. Tacrolimus, which is made in Japan (Prograf; Astellas Pharma, Tokyo, Japan), is an immunosuppressive drug which is one of the common drugs for allogenic organ transplantation in our coun-try and can suppress the immunological reaction in the recipient's immunological reaction and consequently reduces the rejection reaction against the transferred organs [56]. The working mechanisms of tacrolimus are the inhibition of differen-tiation of the lymphocyte reacted to the alloantigens, cytotoxic T cell prolifera-tion, interleukin-2 receptor development, and production of IL-2 and IFN-γ produced from the T cell-derived soluble mediator [57]. The effectiveness of the tacrolimus is well known for the recipients received solid organ transplantation and other diseases due to immunological abnormality like rheumatoid arthritis, which are caused immunological disorder induced T cell reaction [58, 59]. The patients who experienced multiple implantation failures showed elevated Th1 lymphocyte populations, consequently showing high Th1/Th2 cell ratio [1]. Immunological abnormalities are one of the major underlying etiologies for RIF after ART treatment. Recently, we measured the Th1 and Th2 cells and Th1/Th2 cell ratios from the peripheral blood among the patients who experienced RIF for ART treatment. The patients who were greater than 18 and less than 40 years old registered at Sugiyama Clinic, Tokyo, Japan, from September 2014 to March 2016, and 40% of them had elevated Th1/Th2 cell ratios ($\geq$10.3) (Nakagawa K et al., unpublished data). This figure further supports that immunological etiolo-gies can impact the prevalence of RIF.

Currently, we published two prospective cohort studies about using tacrolimus for patients with RIF [60, 61]. A total of 124 RIF women showing increased Th1/Th2 ratios ($\geq$10.3) received immunomodulation treatment by tacrolimus (treatment group). The patients began tacrolimus 1 or 2 days before the ET day and kept receiv-ing it until the check of the pregnancy. The tacrolimus amount per a day varied between 1 and 3 mg due to the values of Th1/Th2 cell ratio (Table 5.2) [60]; women showing a mildly elevated Th1/Th2 ratio ($\geq$10.3 and <13.0) received 1 mg of tacro-limus, daily ($n = 53$). Women showing a moderately elevated Th1/Th2 ratio (>13.0 and <15.8) received 2 mg of tacrolimus, daily ($n = 44$). Women showing a highly

Table 5.2 The daily dose pf tacrolimus was decided depending on the degree of Th1/Th2 elevation

Degree of Th1/Th2 elevation	Daily dose of tacrolimus (mg)
10.3$\leq$ <13.0	1
13.0$\leq$ <15.8	2
15.8<	3

Table 5.3 Reproductive outcomes of the low, middle, and high Th1 groups

	Th1		
	Low	Middle	High
Th1 level	<22.8	22.8≤ <28.8	28.8≤
n	41	41	42
Age, years[a]	35.2	36.4	36.7
Tacrolimus daily dose, mg[a]	1.5	1.9	2.4
Positive hCG, n	23	19	16
Clinical pregnancy, n	20	18	14
Miscarriage, n	1	4	5
Ongoing pregnancy, n	3	5	2
Delivery, n	16	9	7
Ongoing pregnancy/delivery rate, %	46.3	34.1	21.4*

*$p < 0.01$ vs Low group
[a]Mean

elevated Th1/Th2 ratio (>15.8) received 3 mg of tacrolimus daily ($n = 27$). Of 124 patients, 58 women got pregnant (pregnancy rate, 46.8%). In the pregnant group ($n = 58$), 52 women eventually had a clinical pregnancy, which was documented by the detection of GS using ultrasonography (clinical pregnancy rate, 41.9%). Twenty-eight patients delivered healthy babies, and 16 are ongoing (ongoing pregnancy/delivery rate, 35.4%).

Treatment outcome was analyzed based on Th1 cell levels. The 33rd and 66th percentile Th1 cell percentage averages in all patients were 22.8 and 28.8, respectively. According to these values, the women who received tacrolimus were classified into three groups as follows: the patients showing less than 22.8 (Th1 < 22.8) of Th1 cell percentage were classified into the Low group, those showing 22.8 ≤ Th1 < 28.8 of Th1 cell percentage were placed in the Middle group, and those showing more than 28.8 (28.8 ≤ Th1) made up the High group. The hCG-positive rates of the Low, Middle, and High groups were 56.1%, 46.3%, and 38.1%, respectively, and no significant differences were seen among these three groups (Table 5.3). The clinical pregnancy rates (CPRs) for the Low, Middle, and High groups were 48.8%, 43.9%, and 33.3%, respectively. The CPR of the High group was lower than those of the Low and Middle groups; however, this difference was not significant. The miscarriage rate for the Low, Middle, and High groups was 5.0% ($n = 1$), 16.7% ($n = 3$), and 28.6% ($n = 4$), respectively ($P = $ NS). The ongoing/delivery pregnancy rate (≥12 weeks of gestation) of the Low group was 46.3%, which was significantly higher than that of the High group (23.8%, $P = 0.03$) but not different from that of the Middle group (36.6%) (Table 5.2) [61].

Immunological rejection and tolerance in the establishment of pregnancy call for a reconsideration. There is a long-held belief that a fetus and a placenta mount alloreactivity at the maternal-fetal junction. Hence, for the establishment of pregnancy, a pregnant woman should have a decreased cellular immunity to tolerate an invading embryo. The implantation of the transferred embryo to the uterine endometrium begins from both the acceleration of immune tolerance by the dendritic cells (DCs) and regulatory T cells (Treg) and the suppression of immunological rejection by the natural killer (NK) cells and macrophages in the local region (uterine endometrium) [62, 63]. After transient Th1 immunity at the local area, Th1 and Th2 immune responses are balanced locally and systematically. This balance is again shifted to the Th1 immune response at the time of parturition [1].

The Th1/Th2 ratio was developed to reflect the balance between Th1 and Th2 immune responses, and increased Th1/Th2 ratios have been reported in women with RIF [35, 39, 64]. The immunosuppressive treatment has been applied to women with RIF who have increased Th1/ Th2 cell ratios. In the present study, we used the Th1/Th2 cell ratio as an index of implantation failure, but based on our hypothesis mentioned above, we investigated Th1 cell levels as an index for judging the effect of tacrolimus treatment. Therefore, we divided the RIF patients who were treated with tacrolimus into three groups according to the Th1 cell levels (Low, Middle, and High groups). As the Th1 cell percentage increased, the pregnancy rates and clinical pregnancy rates were decreased although statistically insignificant. The ongoing pregnancy rate in the High group was significantly lower than that in the Low group. This may indicate that women with an elevated Th1 cell levels have an inadequate immune tolerance which results in an increased risk of pregnancy losses.

Currently, the daily dosage of tacrolimus treatment is decided depending on the degree of Th1/Th2 elevation, which was calculated using the data of normal women with a history of normal delivery by either natural conception or AIH [11]. The present study demonstrated that Th1 cell percentage alone might have affected the ART results, particularly the ongoing pregnancy rate. Therefore, the patients showing a high Th1 cell percentage (>28.8%) might need an increased dosage of tacrolimus, even though they showed only a moderate Th1/Th2 ratio. Indeed, some cases showed a high Th1 cell percentage but with only moderate Th1/Th2 ratios while being treated with tacrolimus and did not achieve pregnancy, but when these patients were treated with an increased daily dosage of tacrolimus compared with the initial dosage (data not show), a pregnancy was achieved. Therefore, the daily dosage of tacrolimus may be determined by the Th1 cell levels only for the treatment of RIF patients.

We indicated that tacrolimus is quite an effective immunosuppressive agent for the patients with RIF showing elevated Th1/Th2 cell ratios. Moreover, this drug is also effective for the RM patients [65]. However, we have not yet performed RCT of this treatment for the RIF and RM patients. We have to make a plan to do this as soon as possible to obtain the confidence of this treatment.

References

1. Hviid MM, Macklon N. Immune modulation treatments – where is the evidence? Fertil Steril. 2017;107:1284–93.
2. Kwak-Kim JYH, Chung-Bang HS, Ng SC, Ntrivalas EI, Mangubat CP, Beaman KD, et al. Increased T helper 1 cytokine responses by circulating T cells are present in women with recurrent pregnancy losses and in infertile women with multiple implantation failures after IVF. Hum Reprod. 2003;18:767–73.

3. Raghupathy R, Makhseed M, Azizieh F, Hassan N, Al-Azemi M, Al-Shamali E. Maternal Th1- and Th2-type reactivity to placental antigens in normal human pregnancy and unexplained recurrent spontaneous abortions. Cell Immunol. 1999;196:122–30.
4. Moffett A, Shreeve N. First do no harm: uterine natural killer (NK) cells in assisted reproduction. Hum Reprod. 2015;30:1519–25.
5. Chaouat G, Zourbas S, Ostojic S, Lappree-Delage G, Dubanchet S, Ledee N, et al. New insights into maternal-fetal interactions at implantation. Reprod Biomed Online. 2001;2:198–203.
6. Mekinian A, Cohen J, Alijotas-Reig J, Carbillon L, Nicaise-Roland P, Kayem G, et al. Unexplained recurrent miscarriage and recurrent implantation failure: is there a place for immunomodulation? Am J Reprod Immunol. 2016;76:8–28.
7. Robertson SA, Jin M, Yu D, Moldenhauer LM, Davies MJ, Hull ML, et al. Corticosteroid therapy in assisted reproduction—immune suppression is a faulty premise. Hum Reprod. 2016;31:2164–73.
8. Boomsma CM, Kavelaars A, Eijkemans MJC, Lentjes EG, Fauser BCJM, Heijnen CJ, et al. Endometrial secretion analysis identifies a cytokine profile predictive of pregnancy in IVF. Hum Reprod. 2009;24:1427–35.
9. Matsubayashi H, Hosaka T, Sugiyama Y, Suzuki T, Arai T, Kondo A, et al. Increased natural killer-cell activity is associated with infertile women. Am J Reprod Immunol. 2001;46:318–22.
10. Emmer PM, Nelen WL, Steegers EA, Hendriks JC, Veerhoek M, Joosten I. Peripheral natural killer cytotoxicity and CD56(pos)CD16(pos) cells increase during early pregnancy in women with a history of recurrent spontaneous abortion. Hum Reprod. 2000;15:1163–9.
11. King K, Smith S, Chapman M, Sacks G. Detailed analysis of peripheral blood natural killer (NK) cells in women with recurrent miscarriage. Hum Reprod. 2010;25:52–8.
12. Tuckerman E, Mariee N, Prakash A, Li TC, Laird S. Uterine natural killer cells in peri-implantation endometrium from women with repeated implantation failure after IVF. J Reprod Immunol. 2010;87:60–6.
13. Boomsma CM, Keay SD, Macklon NS. Peri-implantation glucocorticoid administration for assisted reproductive technology cycles. Cochrane Database Syst Rev. 2012;6:CD005996.
14. Ando T, Suganuma N, Furuhashi M, Asada Y, Kondo I, Tomoda Y. Successful glucocorticoid treatment for patients with abnormal autoimmunity on in vitro fertilization and embryo transfer. J Assist Reprod Genet. 1996;13:776–81.
15. Bider D, Amoday I, Tur-Kaspa I, Livshits A, Dor J. The addition of a glucocorticoid to the protocol of programmed oocyte retrieval for in-vitro fertilization—a randomized study. Hum Reprod. 1996;11:1606–8.
16. Moffitt D, Queenan JTJ, Veeck LL, Schoolcraft W, Miller CE, Muasher SJ. Low-dose glucocorticoids after in vitro fertilization and embryo transfer have no significant effect on pregnancy rate. Fertil Steril. 1995;63:571–7.
17. Kemeter P, Feichtinger W. Prednisolone supplementation to Clomid and/or gonadotrophin stimulation for in-vitro fertilization—a prospective randomized trial. Hum Reprod. 1986;1:441–4.
18. Kim CH, Chae HD, Kang BM, Chang YS, Mok JE. The immunotherapy during in vitro fertilization and embryo transfer cycles in infertile patients with endometriosis. J Obstet Gynaecol Res. 1997;23:463–70.
19. Ubaldi F, Rienzi L, Ferrero S, Anniballo R, Iacobelli M, Cobellis L, et al. Low dose prednisolone administration in routine ICSI patients does not improve pregnancy and implantation rates. Hum Reprod. 2002;17:1544–7.
20. Tan SL, Balen A, elHussein E, Campbell S, Jacobs HS. The administration of glucocorticoids for the prevention of ovarian hyperstimulation syndrome in in vitro fertilization: a prospective randomized study. Fertil Steril. 1992;58:378–83.
21. Stern C, Chamley L, Hale L, Kloss M, Speirs A, Baker HW. Antibodies to beta2 glycoprotein I are associated with in vitro fertilization implantation failure as well as recurrent miscarriage: results of a prevalence study. Fertil Steril. 1998;70:938–44.
22. Reimand K, Talja I, Metskula K, Kadastik U, Matt K, Uibo R. Autoantibody studies of female patients with reproductive failure. J Reprod Immunol. 2001;51:167–76.

23. Taylor PV, Campbell JM, Scott JS. Presence of autoantibodies in women with unexplained infertility. Am J Obstet Gynecol. 1989;161:377–9.
24. Geva E, Amit A, Lerner-Geva L, Yaron Y, Daniel Y, Schwartz T, et al. Prednisone and aspirin improve pregnancy rate in patients with reproductive failure and autoimmune antibodies: a prospective study. Am J Reprod Immunol. 2000;43:36–40.
25. Taniguchi F. Results of prednisolone given to improve the outcome of in vitro fertilization-embryo transfer in women with antinuclear antibodies. J Reprod Med. 2005;50:383–8.
26. Nelson SM, Greer IA. The potential role of heparin in assisted conception. Hum Reprod Update. 2008;14:623–45.
27. Berker B, Taşkin S, Kahraman K, Taşkin EA, Atabekoglu C, Sonmezer M. The role of low-molecular-weight heparin in recurrent implantation failure: a prospective, quasi-randomized, controlled study. Fertil Steril. 2011;95:2499–502.
28. Fawzy M, El-Refaeey AA. Does combined prednisolone and low molecular weight heparin have a role in unexplained implantation failure? Arch Gynecol Obstet. 2014;289:677–80.
29. Noci I, Milanini MN, Ruggiero M, Papini F, Fuzzi B, Artini PG. Effect of dalteparin sodium administration on IVF outcome in non-thrombophilic young women: a pilot study. Reprod Biomed Online. 2011;22:615–20.
30. Urman B, Ata B, Yakin K, Alatas C, Aksoy S, Mercan R, et al. Luteal phase empirical low molecular weight heparin administration in patients with failed ICSI embryo transfer cycles: a randomized open-labeled pilot trial. Hum Reprod. 2009;24(7):1640.
31. Qublan H, Amarin Z, Dabbas M, Farraj A-E, Beni-Merei Z, Al-Akash H, et al. Low-molecular-weight heparin in the treatment of recurrent IVF-ET failure and thrombophilia: a prospective randomized placebo-controlled trial. Hum Fertil. 2008;11:246–53.
32. Hanevik HI, Friberg M, Bergh A, Haraldsen C, Kahn JA. Do acetyl salicylic acid and terbutaline in combination increase the probability of a clinical pregnancy in patients undergoing IVF/ICSI? J Obstet Gynaecol. 2012;32:786–9.
33. Dirckx K, Cabri P, Merien A, Galajdova L, Gerris J, Dhont M, et al. Does low-dose aspirin improve pregnancy rate in IVF/ICSI? A randomized double-blind placebo controlled trial. Hum Reprod. 2009;24:856–60.
34. Siristatidis CS, Dodd SR, Drakeley AJ. Aspirin for in vitro fertilisation. Cochrane Database Syst Rev. 2011;11:CD004832.
35. Clark DA, Coulam CB, Stricker RBI. Intravenous immunoglobulins (IVIG) efficacious in early pregnancy failure? A critical review and meta-analysis for patients who fail in vitro fertilization and embryo transfer (IVF). J Assist Reprod Genet. 2006;23:1–13.
36. Ruiz JE, Kwak JY, Baum L, Gilman-Sachs A, Beaman KD, Kim YB, et al. Effect of intravenous immunoglobulin G on natural killer cell cytotoxicity in vitro in women with recurrent spontaneous abortion. J Reprod Immunol. 1996;31:125–41.
37. Ramos-Medina R, García-Segovia A, Gil J, Carbone J, Aguarón de la Cruz A, Seyfferth A, et al. Experience in IVIg therapy for selected women with recurrent reproductive failure and NK cell expansion. Am J Reprod Immunol. 2014;71:458–66.
38. Stephenson MD, Fluker MR. Treatment of repeated unexplained in vitro fertilization failure with intravenous immunoglobulin: a randomized, placebo-controlled Canadian trial. Fertil Steril. 2000;74:1108–13.
39. Virro MR, Winger EE, Reed JL. Intravenous immunoglobulin for repeated IVF failure and unexplained infertility. Am J Reprod Immunol. 2012;68:218–25.
40. Winger EE, Reed JL, Ashoush S, El-Toukhy T, Ahuja S, Taranissi M. Elevated preconception CD56 t16 t and/or Th1:Th2 levels predict benefit from IVIG therapy in subfertile women undergoing IVF. Am J Reprod Immunol. 2011;66:394–403.
41. Winger EE, Reed JL, Ashoush S, Ahuja S, El-Toukhy T, Taranissi M. Treatment with adalimumab (Humira) and intravenous immunoglobulin improves pregnancy rates in women undergoing IVF. Am J Reprod Immunol. 2009;61:113–20.
42. Winger EE, Reed JL, Ashoush S, El-Toukhy T, Ahuja S, Taranissi M. Degree of TNF-alpha/IL-10 cytokine elevation correlates with IVF success rates in women undergoing treatment with adalimumab (Humira) and IVIG. Am J Reprod Immunol. 2011;65:610–8.

43. Li J, Chen Y, Liu C, Hu Y, Li L. Intravenous immunoglobulin treatment for repeated IVF/ICSI failure and unexplained infertility: a systematic review and a meta-analysis. Am J Reprod Immunol. 2013;70:434–47.
44. Winger EE, Reed JL, Ashoush S, El-Toukhy T, Taranissi M. Die-off ratio correlates with increased TNF-alpha: IL-10 ratio and decreased IVF success rates correctable with Humira. Am J Reprod Immunol. 2012;68:428–37.
45. Bansal AS, Bajardeen B, Thum MY. The basis and value of currently used immunomodulatory therapies in recurrent miscarriage. J Reprod Immunol. 2012;93:41–51.
46. Clark DA. Intralipid as treatment for recurrent unexplained abortion? Am J Reprod Immunol. 1994;32:290–3.
47. Roussev RG, Acacio B, Ng SC, Coulam CB. Duration of intralipid's suppressive effect on NK cell's functional activity. Am J Reprod Immunol. 2008;60:258–63.
48. Ndukwe G. Recurrent embryo implantation failure after in vitro fertilisation: improved outcome following intralipid infusion in women with elevated T Helper 1 response. Hum Fertil. 2011;14:21–2.
49. El-khayat W, El Sadek M. Intralipid for repeated implantation failure (RIF): a randomized controlled trial. Fertil Steril. 2015;104:e26.
50. Dakhly DMR, Bayoumi YA, Sharkawy M, Allah SHG, Hassan MA, Gouda HM, et al. Intralipid supplementation in women with recurrent spontaneous abortion and elevated levels of natural killer cells. Int J Gynecol Obstet. 2016;135:324–7.
51. Chaouat G, Ledee-Bataille N, Dubanchet S, Zourbas S, Sandra O, Martal J. Th1/Th2 paradigm in pregnancy: paradigm lost? Int Arch Allergy Immunol. 2004;134:93–119.
52. Saito S, Nakashima A, Shima T, Ito M. Th1/Th2/Th17 and regulatory T-cell paradigm in pregnancy. Am J Reprod Immunol. 2010;63:601–10.
53. Ng SC, Gilman-Sachs A, Thakar P, Beaman KD, Beer AE, Kwak-Kim J. Expression of intracellular Th1 and Th2 cytokines in women with recurrent spontaneous abortion, implantation failures after IVF-ET or normal pregnancy. Am J Reprod Immunol. 2002;48:77–86.
54. Riley JK. Trophoblast immune receptors in maternal-fetal tolerance. Immunol Investig. 2008;37:395–426.
55. Goring SM, Lew AR, Ghement I, Kasekar A, Eyaow O, L'italien GJ, Kasiske B. A network meta-analysis of the efficacy of belatacept, cyclosporine and tacrolimus for immunosuppression therapy in adult renal transplant recipients. Curr Med Res Opin. 2014;30:1473–87.
56. Uchida K. Long-term Prograf multicenter retrospective study in kidney transplantation: seven-year follow-up. Transplant Now. 2006;19:380–9.
57. Kino T, Hatanaka H, Miyata S, Inamura N, Nishiyama M, Yajima T, Goto T, Okuhara M, Kohsaka M, Aoki H, Ohiai T. FK-506, a novel immunosuppressant isolated from a Streptomyces. II. Immunosuppressive effect of FK-506 in vitro. J Antibiot. 1987;40:1256–65.
58. Ram R, Gafter-Gvili A, Yeshuru M, Paul M, Raanani P, Shpilberg O. Prophylaxis regimens for GVHD: systematic review and metaanalysis. Bone Marrow Transplant. 2009;43:643–53.
59. Ramiro S, Gaujoux-Viala C, Nam JL, Smolen JS, Buch M, Gossec L, van der Heijde D, Winthrop K, Landewé R. Safety of synthetic and biological DMARDs: a systematic literature review informing the 2013 update of the EULAR recommendations for management of rheumatoid arthritis. Ann Rheum Dis. 2014;73:529–35.
60. Nakagawa K, Kwak-Kim J, Ota K, Hisano M, Sugiyama R, Yamaguchi K. Immunosuppression with Tacrolimus improved reproductive outcome of women with repeated implantation failure and elevated peripheral blood Th1/Th2 cell ratios. Am J Reprod Immunol. 2015;73:353–61.
61. Nakagawa K, Kwak-Kim J, Kuroda K, Sugiyama R, Yamaguchi K. Immunosuppressive treatment using tacrolimus promotes pregnancy outcome in infertile women with repeated implantation failures. Am J Reprod Immunol. 2017. https://doi.org/10.1111/aji.12682.
62. Saito S, Shima T, Nakashima A, Inada K, Yoshino O. Role of paternal antigen-specific Treg cells in successful implantation. Am J Reprod Immunol. 2016;75:310–6.
63. Than NG, Romero R, Erez O, et al. Emergence of hormonal and redox regulation of galectin-1 in placental mammals: implication in maternal-fetal immune tolerance. Proc Natl Acad Sci U S A. 2008;105:15819–24.

64. Graphou O, Chioti A, Pantazi A, et al. Effect of intravenous immunoglobulin treatment on the Th1/Th2 balance in women with recurrent spontaneous abortions. Am J Reprod Immunol. 2003;49:21–9.
65. Nakagawa K, Kuroda K, Sugiyama R, Yamaguchi K. After 12 consecutive miscarriages, a patient received immunosuppressive treatment and delivered an infant. Reprod Med Biol. 2017. https://doi.org/10.1002/rmb2.12040.

Chapter 6
Unexplained Infertility: Treatment Strategy for Unexplained Infertility

Keiji Kuroda and Asako Ochiai

Abstract The candidate causes of unexplained infertility are (1) oviduct dysfunction with tubal patency, (2) fertilization failure and (3) implantation failure without an organic lesion. At any rate, undetectable causes of infertility inhibit the processes of sperm-egg encounter or implantation. Thus, patients with unexplained infertility cannot benefit from general infertility treatment, including timed intercourse or intrauterine insemination. Assisted reproductive technology including in vitro fertilization can overcome tubal dysfunction and fertilization failure, but not recurrent implantation failure (RIF). As regards RIF, hysteroscopy and blood tests for immunological abnormality and recurrent miscarriage should be performed as clinically practicable implantation testing. The treatment of RIF is the remedy of detected causes. If there is no cause of implantation failure, treatment approaches include endometrial injury during luteal phase, systemic single-dose G-CSF injection at embryo transfer, a vitrified-warmed single blastocyst transfer with assisted hatching and hyaluronan-enriched medium.

Keywords Unexplained infertility · Fertilization failure · Tubal dysfunction Recurrent implantation failure · Immune infertility · Implantation testing Endometrial injury

6.1 Treatment Strategy for Unexplained Infertility

Unsuccessful pregnancy without specific reasons identified is stressful and frustrating for infertile couples as well as gynaecologists. Unexplained infertility occurs in 15–30% of infertility patients, who are likely to fail to conceive due to undetected

K. Kuroda (✉)
Center for Reproductive Medicine and Implantation Research, Sugiyama Clinic Shinjuku,
Tokyo, Japan

Department of Obstetrics and Gynaecology, Faculty of Medicine, Juntendo University,
Tokyo, Japan
e-mail: arthur@juntendo.ac.jp

A. Ochiai
Department of Obstetrics and Gynaecology, Faculty of Medicine, Juntendo University,
Tokyo, Japan

© Springer Nature Singapore Pte Ltd. 2018
K. Kuroda et al. (eds.), *Treatment Strategy for Unexplained Infertility and
Recurrent Miscarriage*, https://doi.org/10.1007/978-981-10-8690-8_6

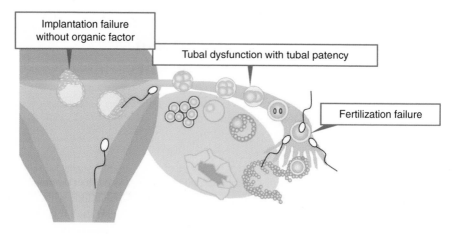

Fig. 6.1 Causes of infertility in unexplained infertility. The candidate causes of unexplained infertility are (1) oviduct dysfunction with tubal patency, (2) fertilization failure and (3) implantation failure

Table 6.1 Data in unexplained infertility

• Proportion of unexplained infertility in infertile couples: 15–30%
• Cumulative pregnancy rate by general non-ART fertility treatment or expectant management: 10–20%
(Clinical pregnancy rate: <5% per month)
• Cumulative pregnancy rate by general fertility treatment with superovulation using gonadotropins: 50–60%
(Multiple pregnancy rate: 6–35%)
(Clinical pregnancy rate: 20% per month)
• Cumulative pregnancy rate after laparoscopic surgery: 20–30%
(Clinical pregnancy rate: 6% per month)

causes after basic fertility investigations. The candidate causes of unexplained infertility are (1) oviduct dysfunction with tubal patency, including gamete and embryo transport disorder and oocyte retrieval failure at the tube fimbria, (2) fertilization failure and (3) implantation failure without an organic lesion (Fig. 6.1). At any rate, undetectable causes of infertility inhibit the processes of encounter of the sperm and egg or implantation after fertilization. Thus, patients with unexplained infertility cannot benefit from general infertility treatment, including timed intercourse or intrauterine insemination (IUI). The cumulative pregnancy rate by general infertility treatment is 10–20% in unexplained infertility patients, which is comparable to that of expectant management [1, 2] (Table 6.1). When proceeding to in vitro fertilization (IVF), the reasons for unexplained infertility sometimes are revealed. Therefore, timed intercourse or IUI should not be repeated discursively. IVF or intracytoplasmic sperm injection (ICSI) can overcome tubal dysfunction and fertilization failure. In patients with unexplained infertility, gynaecologists must explain the reasons why patients cannot conceive and discuss active infertility treatment, including assisted reproductive technology (ART) (for details of the undetected causes of unexplained infertility, refer to the Chap. 1).

6.1.1 Superovulation with Gonadotropins and IUI

Regarding outcomes of non-ART infertility treatment in unexplained infertility, there is no significant difference in pregnancy rates achieved with mild ovarian stimulation using clomiphene citrate or an aromatase inhibitor. However, according to some reviews, the cumulative pregnancy rate after combination treatment of superovulation with gonadotropins and IUI was 50–60% [1, 2] (Fig. 6.2, Table 6.1). Presumably, a large number of sperms and eggs after superovulation and IUI may solve the problems of oviduct dysfunction or endometriosis in patients with unexplained infertility. Some reviews demonstrated that ovarian hyperstimulation syndrome did not occur at high rates; however the incidence of multiple pregnancies is as high as 6–35% [1, 2]. We have to inform the risk of multiple pregnancies to the patients before starting ovarian stimulation.

6.1.2 Laparoscopic Surgery

Normal findings of hysterosalpingography do not denote normal tubal function. To our knowledge, no examination exists to determine whether the oviducts function in oocyte pickup at the tube fimbria or transportation of gametes and embryos by ciliated epithelial cells. These problems with tubal function inhibit the process of

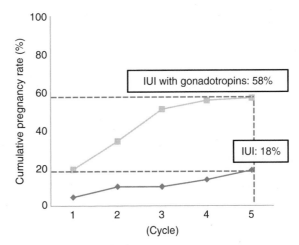

Fig. 6.2 Pregnancy rate of combination treatment of superovulation and intrauterine insemination. The cumulative pregnancy rate after combination treatment of superovulation with gonadotropins and IUI was significantly higher at 50–60% than that of only IUI at 10–20% in the patients with unexplained infertility. IUI: intrauterine insemination. Chaffkin ML, et al., Fertil Steril. 1991

IUI: intrauterine insemination

Fig. 6.3 Pregnancy rate after laparoscopic surgery. Randomized controlled trial of laparoscopic surgery for the patients with unexplained infertility demonstrates 30% of cumulative pregnancy rates after laparoscopic resection of mild endometriosis and 18% of that after diagnostic laparoscopy only. Marcoux S, et al., N Engl JMed. 1997

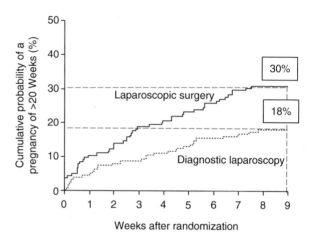

sperm-egg encounter. In 20–70% of infertile couples with normal hysterosalpingography findings, laparoscopy reveals abnormal intrapelvic findings, including peritubal adhesion and endometriosis [3]. Endometriosis induces intrapelvic chronic inflammatory changes, resulting in suppression of sperm mobility, fertilization and embryo development [4]. If undetectable infertile causes, such as early stage endometriosis or peritubal adhesion, were detected and treated laparoscopically, some women might achieve a pregnancy. However, the outcomes after laparoscopic surgery demonstrate only 6% and 20–30% monthly and cumulative pregnancy rates, respectively [3, 5] (Fig. 6.3). If no specific finding is recognized during laparoscopy, the infertile couples should switch treatment to IVF.

6.1.3 In Vitro Fertilization

In conventional IVF, the fertilization rate for collected matured oocytes and concentration controlled sperms is generally 60–80%. One of the undetected causes of infertility is fertilization failure, which cannot be revealed without proceeding to IVF. Most patients with a history of fertilization failure by conventional IVF can achieve a pregnancy after ICSI. However, complete fertilization failure occurs in 1–5% of couples after ICSI [6, 7]. These patients may have a problem with oocyte activation, which is a repetitive transient intracytoplasmic Ca^{2+} increase (Ca^{2+} oscillations) at fertilization. Oocyte activation failure, including post-fertilized cleavage arrest and polyspermy, is also a cause of unexplained infertility [6]. Some patients with oocyte activation failure require ICSI in combination with assisted oocyte activation (AOA), which is the procedure to increase Ca^{2+} concentration in the oocyte. AOA includes electrical and chemical activation using calcium ionophore, puromycin or strontium chloride. However, an increase in intracellular Ca^{2+} level after AOA is completely different from Ca^{2+} oscillations after IVF or ICSI [8]. Sperm-specific protein, phospholipase C zeta (PLCζ), is a strong candidate sperm factor. PLCζ RNA injection can induce similar Ca^{2+} oscillations to that after IVF. Thus, PLCζ may become useful as a clinical application for egg activation failure in the future [6, 8].

6.2 Examination and Diagnosis of Implantation Failure

At implantation, a fertilized egg at the tubal ampulla develops into a blastocyst and reaches the uterine cavity. On the other hand, in response to elevated circulating progesterone levels after ovulation, the uterine endometrium is morphologically and functionally changed into decidualizing endometrial cells. This process forms the optimal window of implantation (WOI). The blastocyst shed from the zona pellucida and decidual endometrium crosstalk mutually, leading to completion of implantation through the processes of apposition, attachment, adhesion and encapsulation. Successful pregnancy requires endometrial receptivity, embryo competency and their reciprocal crosstalk.

6.2.1 Diagnosis of Recurrent Implantation Failure

Preimplantation genetic screening (PGS), which is embryo chromosomal testing, has been increasingly common worldwide. Yet, a selected chromosomally normal embryo does not yield all implantation failure. More than 30% of patients with a history of recurrent implantation failure (RIF) cannot achieve a live birth even with use of PGS [9, 10]. Most reports of definitions of RIF describe two or three or more failed treatment cycles [11]. According to Japanese ART data in 2014, the clinical pregnancy rate of 30-year-old women is 42%, including miscarriage, resulting in an 89% cumulative pregnancy rate after four embryo transfers (Table 6.2) [12]. This

Table 6.2 Number of embryo transfer and cumulative implantation rates based on age

Age (years)	Implantation rate (/embryo transfer)	No of embryo transfer (times)			
		2	3	4	5
25–30	42.0%	66.4%	80.5%	88.7%	93.4%
32	40.5%	64.6%	78.9%	87.5%	92.5%
34	38.7%	62.4%	77.0%	85.9%	91.3%
36	36.3%	59.4%	74.2%	83.5%	89.5%
38	32.1%	53.9%	68.7%	78.7%	85.6%
40	24.8%	43.4%	57.5%	68.0%	76.0%
42	17.7%	32.3%	44.3%	54.1%	62.2%
44	10.7%	20.3%	28.8%	36.4%	43.2%
45–	6.0%	11.6%	16.9%	21.9%	26.6%

Cumulative implantation rate: blue flame; >50%, red flame; >80%
Japan Society of Obstetrics and Gynecology, ART data book, 2014

means that the remaining 11% of women still may not conceive accidentally. Therefore, the diagnosis of RIF, depending on patient age, requires four or more embryo transfer cycles with morphologically good embryos. Reproductive physicians must recommend examinations for implantation failure and discuss the therapeutic strategy before pursuing embryo transfer in the same way.

6.2.2 Examination of Implantation Failure

Intrauterine fibroids and polyps inhibit implantation, and they are diagnosable and treatable. However, some infertile patients with a history of RIF have no organic uterine abnormality. The causes of implantation failure are problems with the uterine cavity, embryo, crosstalk between the uterus and an embryo and immune rejection against an embryo.

The problem of crosstalk currently is in the research stage [13]. Thus, it is impossible to assess its use in clinical practice. It is difficult to solve the problems with the uterine cavity or embryo by non-ART infertility treatment. Therefore, patients with implantation failure should be treated appropriately using ART. Implantation testing is shown in Table 6.3. Examinations of the uterus include hysteroscopy for local intrauterine circumstance and identification of the WOI by endometrial receptivity array (ERA®) or nucleolar channel system (NCS). Hysteroscopy and ultrasonography can identify an undetectable disorder, such as chronic endometritis (CE), intrauterine adhesion and small endometrial polyps. ERA® is the tool to identify individual optimal WOI, based on 238 genes identified from microarray analysis of decidualizing human endometrium [14]. This is a novel and effective, but expensive, test offered by a Spanish company, IGENOMIX (available in the public domain at http://www.igenomix.com/tests/endometrial-receptivity-test-era/). NCS are membranous organelles of epithelial cell nuclei, which appear briefly during WOI [15].

Table 6.3 Implantation testing

Intrauterine circumstance and window of implantation
- Hysteroscopy
- ERA® (Endometrial receptivity array)
- NCS (Nucleolar channel system)

Immunological test
- Th1/Th2 cell level
- Serum NK cell activity
- 25OH vitamin D (Storage form)

Examination of embryo
- Preimplantation genetic screening

Examination for recurrent miscarriage
- Reference of introduction in unexplained recurrent miscarriage

Underline: general clinical applicable tests

Thus, the immunostaining of NCS also may be used to confirm personal WOI as a future clinical application. The maternal immunological tests against semi-allograft embryos include T-helper (Th)1/Th2 cell level, serum natural killer (NK) cell activity and serum 25-hydroxyvitamin D_3 (25OHVD) as an immunological regulator. The examination of an embryo is only PGS as a chromosomal test. The risk factors for recurrent miscarriage, including thrombophilia and thyroid disorder, are relatively highly prevalent in patients with a history of RIF [16–18]. If not examined with the test, patients with RIF may suffer miscarriage after finally achieving implantation. Therefore, we recommend examinations for recurrent miscarriage at the same time as implantation testing (for details, refer to Chap. 7). Taken together, hysteroscopy and blood tests for immunological abnormality and recurrent miscarriage should be performed as clinically practicable implantation testing. The therapeutic strategy for RIF should be discussed according to the results of the tests.

6.3 Treatment of Implantation Failure

Treatment of RIF after implantation testing is shown in Table 6.4. The standard treatment is to identify and address the cause of unsuccessful implantation. We demonstrated the treatment for the uterus, embryo, immunity and timing of implantation.

Table 6.4 Treatment of repeated implantation failure

For uterus
- Chronic endometritis: antibiotics; 1. doxycycline, 2. ciprofloxacin + metronidazole
- Endometrial polyp: hysteroscopic surgery
- Cesarian scar syndrome: hysteroscopic surgery (+ laparoscopic surgery)
- Endometrial injury
- Intrauterine G-CSF injection
- Progesterone treatment

For embryo
- Blastocyst culture
- Single embryo transfer
- Assisted hatching
- Hyaluronan-enriched embryo transfer medium (Preimplantation genetic screening)

For immunity
- Th1/Th2 cell ratio: tacrolimus, adalimumab, vitamin D, progesterone
- NK cell activity: vitamin D, progesterone
- 25OH vitamin D: vitamin D

For timing of implantation
- Change of embryo transfer timing
- Vitrified-warmed embryo transfer

6.3.1 Treatment of an Embryo

When a pregnancy test is negative after transferring a cleavage embryo, we cannot identify the reason for unsuccessful implantation, whether it is cleavage arrest or implantation failure. Therefore, the embryo should be cultivated until the blastocyst stage. We also recommend zona pellucida incision by assisted hatching and dip treatment in an embryo transfer medium rich in hyaluronan, which enhances the attachment between an embryo and uterine endometrium, as supportive procedures of implantation. The use of assisted hatching and hyaluronan-enriched medium at embryo transfer is beneficial for some RIF patients [19, 20].

There have been some reports of an adverse effect of a poor-quality embryo on implantation [21, 22]. Therefore, the implantation rate after double embryo transfer, including a poor-quality embryo, is lower than that after elective single embryo transfer [23]. Therefore, multiple embryo transfer is not recommended for patients with a history of RIF.

6.3.2 Control of Implantation Site

Optimization of intrauterine circumstance is important for implantation. Hysteroscopy often shows CE and micropolyps in RIF patients. A local inflammatory disease, CE is found in approximately 30–60% of women with a history of RIF [24–26]. When it is suspected, CE is diagnosed by immunostaining with the plasmacyte marker, CD138, of biopsied endometrial samples. The responsible microorganisms of CE include a wide variety, such as *Escherichia coli*, *Enterococcus*, *Streptococcus*, *Mycoplasma* and *Chlamydia trachomatis* [26]. Some endometrium with CE demonstrates only plasmacytes without bacteria detection [24, 26]. Thus, the recommended treatment for patients with CE is broad-spectrum antibiotics: oral doxycycline 100 mg twice a day for 2 weeks as a first choice and a combination of ciprofloxacin 500 mg/metronidazole 500 mg twice a day for 2 weeks as a second choice [24] (for details, refer to Chap. 4).

Regarding endometrial polyps, polyps detected in the uterine cavity should be excised by hysteroscopic surgery in patients with a history of RIF. In particular, polyps located at the uterotubal junction are strongly associated with infertility. Therefore, such polyps should be removed, even if they are micropolyps [27]. Some micropolyps arise from CE. Then, antibiotics should be administered preoperatively.

In infertile women with a symptom of abnormal bleeding and a prior delivery by caesarean section, bloody fluid from the caesarean scar defect often prohibits implantation, leading to infertility (caesarean scar syndrome). The bloody fluid derived from the caesarean scar defect may flow into the uterine cavity, resulting in implantation failure. To identify a caesarean scar defect, transvaginal ultrasound demonstrates bloody fluid retention in the uterine cavity from menstruation to ovulation. Furthermore, confirmation of dendritic vessels and erythrogenic scar on hysteroscopic findings is an important information for diagnosis. Recent standard treatment is hysteroscopic surgery. If the residual myometrial caesarean scar is extremely thin, the scar should be resected and sutured laparoscopically [28] (for details, refer to Chap. 4).

Other treatments for RIF include progesterone therapy. Impaired decidualization of the endometrium is associated with infertility as well as miscarriage [29]. Progesterone can regulate decidual change of the uterine endometrium and maternal immune tolerance for implantation [30].

Endometrial injury is one of the treatments for RIF. According to basic research, the mechanism of improvement of endometrial receptivity by endometrial injury may be induction of an inflammatory reaction for implantation, promotion of decidualization of endometrial stromal cells and activation of endometrial stem cells during the wound-healing process [31, 32]. No effect of local injury to the endometrium on implantation in patients without a history of RIF (three or more embryo transfer failures) was reported, although all results demonstrated no adverse influence on implantation rate [33]. This suggests that we can carry out endometrial injury if the patients with infertility are suspected of having RIF. The procedure for endometrial injury is to simply perform endometrial sampling by a Pipelle endometrial biopsy sampler at approximately 7 days before initiation of menstruation (Fig. 6.4). Endometrial injury during the luteal phase in a previous cycle of embryo transfer is basically recommended; thus, we must advise all patients to protect intercourse during the cycle of endometrial injury [34]. Endometrial injury at the same time as oocyte retrieval is not recommended.

The effectiveness of intrauterine hCG infusion and systemic subcutaneous or local infusion of G-CSF has been reported recently. The use of hCG and G-CSF may induce decidualization of the endometrium and regulate immune tolerance at implantation. Administration of G-CSF for RIF remains controversial. The trials suggested that systemic administration of G-CSF, but not hCG infusion, improves pregnancy outcomes, in patients with RIF [35, 36]. Combination treatment of systemic G-CSF injection and CD133[+] cells isolated from peripheral blood via intra-arterial catheterization was reported as a treatment for RIF, including in patients with Asherman's syndrome and endometrial atrophy. This autologous cell therapy improved endometrial thickness, leading to successful pregnancy in patients with intractable implantation failure [37]. This treatment has just been started; thus, further investigations are needed to be applied to a clinical application.

6.3.3 Optimization of Window of Implantation

Successful implantation needs synchronous development of a competent embryo and decidualizing endometrium. Controlled ovarian stimulation for multiple follicle development adversely affects endometrial receptivity, due to the impact of supraphysiologic levels of endocrine abnormality on the proliferative and decidualizing process of the endometrium [38]. It is important to select a freeze-all policy and frozen embryo transfer, not fresh embryo transfer, for management of the optimal WOI. When determining ERA® analysis or NCS, we can confirm whether the

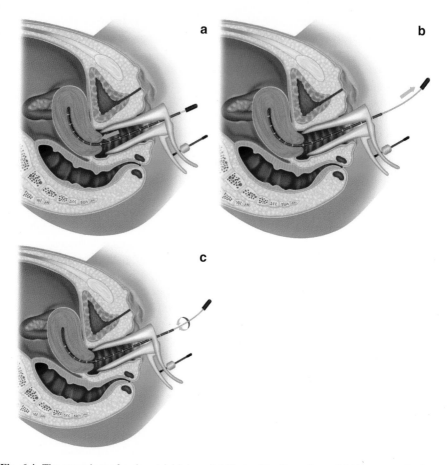

Fig. 6.4 The procedure of endometrial injury. (**a**) First, a Pipelle endometrial biopsy sampler is inserted into the uterine fundus. (**b**) The inner plunger is extracted to apply a sucking force to the endometrial cavity. (**c**) The superficial endometrium is scratched with combining an in-and-out and rotational movement by the Pipelle biopsy sampler several times

uterine endometrium is at optimal timing of implantation. If the result of the ERA® test or NCS is 'nonreceptive', we must validate the optimal WOI with a second test and reschedule the timing of embryo transfer (for details, refer to Chap. 4).

6.3.4 Regulation of Immune Tolerance

Implantation and maintenance of pregnancy requires survival of the semi-allogenic embryo under maternal immune response, such as NK cells, lymphocytes Th1/Th2 cell as well as Th17/regulatory T-cell balance. We focused on the Th1/Th2 cell ratio,

NK cell activity and 25OHVD in implantation testing as a clinical evidence-based approach. Successful pregnancy is involved in balancing of Th1 (interleukin [IL]-2, intracellular interferon [IFN]-γ, and tumour necrosis factor [TNF]-α production) and Th2 (IL-4, IL-5 and IL-10 production) cell ratio in favour of Th2 cells [39, 40]. Impaired Th1/Th2 cell balance, in particular elevated Th1 cell levels, causes reproductive failure, including implantation failure and miscarriage [41, 42]. In the treatment of patients with RIF and an aberrant high Th1/Th2 cell ratio, the use of the Th1 cell-produced cytokine, TNF-α-targeted drug, adalimumab (Humira®), which is an antirheumatic drug, results in good pregnancy outcomes [43]. The certificate of safety compliance of adalimumab treatment remains insufficient, but no increased risk of congenital malformations was reported [44]. Intravenous immunoglobulin (IVIg) also can improve pregnancy outcome by IVF [43]. However, the treatment is extremely expensive in general. Recently, a positive effect of the immunosuppressive drug, tacrolimus (Prograf®), on IVF treatment has been reported in patients with RIF and an elevated Th1/Th2 cell ratio [41]. The use of tacrolimus during pregnancy was reported at no elevated risk of foetal malformation in women who received an organ transplant, including uterus transplantation [45, 46]. Therefore, adalimumab and tacrolimus are expected as novel treatments for RIF patients with immune abnormality.

Regarding NK cells, the relationship of peripheral or uterine NK cells and infertility remains uncertain [47]. In any case, direct immunotherapy for increased NK cells includes prednisolone; however it may inhibit the important inflammatory reaction at implantation. The benefit of prednisolone on implantation failure was not verified [48]. Progesterone therapy suppresses elevated NK cells, induces Th2 cell production and promotes decidualization of the human endometrium [30]. Thus, progesterone would be a better treatment for implantation failure with aberrant high cytotoxic NK cell activity than prednisolone. Vitamin D modulates immune function of helper T cells and NK cell activity. Thus, vitamin D deficiency is associated with infertility as well as pregnancy complications, including miscarriage and pre-eclampsia [49]. In the infertile patients with vitamin D deficiency, low implantation rates after embryo transfer in an oocyte donation programme were reported [50]. The patients with RIF and vitamin D deficiency must take vitamin D supplementation until the ideal 25OHVD serum level of 30 ng/mL is achieved [51] (for details, refer to Chap. 5).

6.3.5 Treatment Strategy for Recurrent Implantation Failure

The treatment protocol for RIF is shown in Fig. 6.5. The cornerstone of treatment is the remedy of detected causes by implantation testing. If no reason for implantation failure is recognized, treatment approaches include (1) local endometrial injury at 7 days before menstruation and (2) systemic single-dose G-CSF injection at subsequent embryo transfer. We also recommend (3) selecting one good-quality blastocyst (or chromosomal normal blastocyst after PGS) and (4) transferring a

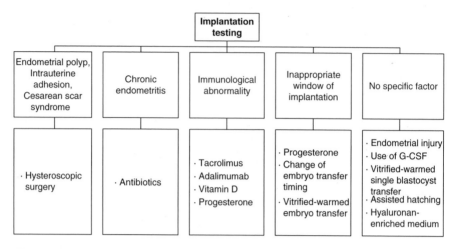

Fig. 6.5 Treatment of recurrent implantation failure. The treatment of recurrent implantation failure is the remedy of detected causes by implantation testing. If there is no cause of implantation failure, treatment approaches include endometrial injury during luteal phase, systemic single-dose G-CSF injection at embryo transfer, a vitrified-warmed single blastocyst transfer with assisted hatching and hyaluronan-enriched medium

vitrified-warmed single blastocyst into the uterus, not fresh cycle and not cleavage stage embryo transfer for regulation of optimal WOI and endometrial receptivity. Furthermore, embryo transfer in combination with (5) assisted hatching and (6) hyaluronan-enriched medium would improve the implantation rate.

If the risk factors for miscarriage were found, treatment is important for protection of pregnancy loss. Regarding thrombophilia, the use of low-dose aspirin is recommended. Note that aspirin not only has anticoagulative action, it also has an anti-inflammatory effect; thus, aspirin treatment may inhibit inflammatory reaction related to implantation [52]. The effect of aspirin treatment on implantation rate was not proven [53–55]. Therefore, aspirin treatment should be initiated from the post-implantation period, at least 7 days after ovulation. Impaired thyroid function and thyroid autoimmunity are associated with an adverse effect on fertility, including folliculogenesis, fertilization, embryo development and implantation [56, 57]. Preconception thyroid disorder must be treated before embryo transfer, even if there is subclinical hypothyroidism.

References

1. Gunn DD, Bates GW. Evidence-based approach to unexplained infertility: a systematic review. Fertil Steril. 2016;105:1566–1574.e1.
2. Chaffkin LM, Nulsen JC, Luciano AA, Metzger DA. A comparative analysis of the cycle fecundity rates associated with combined human menopausal gonadotropin (hMG) and intrauterine insemination (IUI) versus either hMG or IUI alone**presented in part at the 45th

annual meeting of the American Fertility Society, San Francisco, California, November 13 to 16, 1989. Fertil Steril. 1991;55:252–7.

3. Tanahatoe SJ, Hompes PGA, Lambalk CB. Investigation of the infertile couple – should diagnostic laparoscopy be performed in the infertility work up programme in patients undergoing intrauterine insemination? Hum Reprod. 2003;18:8–11.

4. Harada T, Iwabe T, Terakawa N. Role of cytokines in endometriosis. Fertil Steril. 2001;76:1–10.

5. Marcoux S, Maheux R, Berube S, Langevin M, Graves G, Wrixon W, et al. Laparoscopic surgery in infertile, women with minimal or mild endometriosis. N Engl J Med. 1997;337:217–22.

6. Kashir J, Heindryckx B, Jones C, De Sutter P, Parrington J, Coward K. Oocyte activation, phospholipase C zeta and human infertility. Hum Reprod Update. 2010;16:690–703.

7. Flaherty SP, Payne D, Matthews CD. Fertilization failures and abnormal fertilization after intracytoplasmic sperm injection. Hum Reprod. 1998;13:155–64.

8. Yamaguchi T, Ito M, Kuroda K, Takeda S, Tanaka A. The establishment of appropriate methods for egg-activation by human PLCZ1 RNA injection into human oocyte. Cell Calcium. 2017;65:22–30.

9. Scott RT. Introduction: Subchromosomal abnormalities in preimplantation embryonic aneuploidy screening. Fertil Steril. 2017;107:4–5.

10. Treff NR, Franasiak JM. Detection of segmental aneuploidy and mosaicism in the human preimplantation embryo: technical considerations and limitations. Fertil Steril. 2017;107:27–31.

11. Polanski LT, Baumgarten MN, Quenby S, Brosens J, Campbell BK, Raine-Fenning NJ. What exactly do we mean by 'recurrent implantation failure'? A systematic review and opinion. Reprod Biomed Online. 2014;28:409–23.

12. Irahara M, Kuwahara A, Iwasa T, Ishikawa T, Ishihara O, Kugu K, et al. Assisted reproductive technology in Japan: a summary report of 1992–2014 by the Ethics Committee, Japan Society of Obstetrics and Gynecology. Reprod Med Biol. 2017;16:126–32.

13. Altmae S, Reimand J, Hovatta O, Zhang P, Kere J, Laisk T, et al. Research resource: interactome of human embryo implantation: identification of gene expression pathways, regulation, and integrated regulatory networks. Mol Endocrinol. 2012;26:203–17.

14. Diaz-Gimeno P, Horcajadas JA, Martinez-Conejero JA, Esteban FJ, Alama P, Pellicer A, et al. A genomic diagnostic tool for human endometrial receptivity based on the transcriptomic signature. Fertil Steril. 2011;95:50–60.

15. Guffanti E, Kittur N, Brodt ZN, Polotsky AJ, Kuokkanen SM, Heller DS, et al. Nuclear pore complex proteins mark the implantation window in human endometrium. J Cell Sci. 2008;121:2037–45.

16. Mekinian A, Cohen J, Alijotas-Reig J, Carbillon L, Nicaise-Roland P, Kayem G, et al. Unexplained recurrent miscarriage and recurrent implantation failure: is there a place for immunomodulation? Am J Reprod Immunol. 2016;76:8–28.

17. Grandone E, Colaizzo D, Lo Bue A, Checola MG, Cittadini E, Margaglione M. Inherited thrombophilia and in vitro fertilization implantation failure. Fertil Steril. 2001;76:201–2.

18. Azem F, Many A, Ben Ami I, Yovel I, Amit A, Lessing JB, et al. Increased rates of thrombophilia in women with repeated IVF failures. Hum Reprod. 2004;19:368–70.

19. Friedler S, Schachter M, Strassburger D, Esther K, Ron El R, Raziel A. A randomized clinical trial comparing recombinant hyaluronan/recombinant albumin versus human tubal fluid for cleavage stage embryo transfer in patients with multiple IVF-embryo transfer failure. Hum Reprod. 2007;22:2444–8.

20. Martins WP, Rocha IA, Ferriani RA, Nastri CO. Assisted hatching of human embryos: a systematic review and meta-analysis of randomized controlled trials. Hum Reprod Update. 2011;17:438–53.

21. Brosens JJ, Salker MS, Teklenburg G, Nautiyal J, Salter S, Lucas ES, et al. Uterine selection of human embryos at implantation. Sci Rep. 2014;4:3894.

22. Teklenburg G, Salker M, Molokhia M, Lavery S, Trew G, Aojanepong T, et al. Natural selection of human embryos: decidualizing endometrial stromal cells serve as sensors of embryo quality upon implantation. PLoS One. 2010;5:e10258.

23. Wintner EM, Hershko-Klement A, Tzadikevitch K, Ghetler Y, Gonen O, Wintner O, et al. Does the transfer of a poor quality embryo together with a good quality embryo affect the In Vitro Fertilization (IVF) outcome? J Ovarian Res. 2017;10:2.
24. Johnston-MacAnanny EB, Hartnett J, Engmann LL, Nulsen JC, Sanders MM, Benadiva CA. Chronic endometritis is a frequent finding in women with recurrent implantation failure after in vitro fertilization. Fertil Steril. 2010;93:437–41.
25. Kitaya K, Tada Y, Taguchi S, Funabiki M, Hayashi T, Nakamura Y. Local mononuclear cell infiltrates in infertile patients with endometrial macropolyps versus micropolyps. Hum Reprod. 2012;27:3474–80.
26. Kitaya K, Matsubayashi H, Yamaguchi K, Nishiyama R, Takaya Y, Ishikawa T, et al. Chronic endometritis: potential cause of infertility and obstetric and neonatal complications. Am J Reprod Immunol. 2016;75:13–22.
27. Yanaihara A, Yorimitsu T, Motoyama H, Iwasaki S, Kawamura T. Location of endometrial polyp and pregnancy rate in infertility patients. Fertil Steril. 2008;90:180–2.
28. Tanimura S, Funamoto H, Hosono T, Shitano Y, Nakashima M, Ametani Y, et al. New diagnostic criteria and operative strategy for cesarean scar syndrome: endoscopic repair for secondary infertility caused by cesarean scar defect. J Obstet Gynaecol Res. 2015;41:1363–9.
29. Gellersen B, Brosens JJ. Cyclic decidualization of the human endometrium in reproductive health and failure. Endocr Rev. 2014;35:851–905.
30. Szekeres-Bartho J, Balasch J. Progestagen therapy for recurrent miscarriage. Hum Reprod Update. 2008;14:27–35.
31. Gnainsky Y, Granot I, Aldo PB, Barash A, Or Y, Schechtman E, et al. Local injury of the endometrium induces an inflammatory response that promotes successful implantation. Fertil Steril. 2010;94:2030–6.
32. Barash A, Dekel N, Fieldust S, Segal I, Schechtman E, Granot I. Local injury to the endometrium doubles the incidence of successful pregnancies in patients undergoing in vitro fertilization. Fertil Steril. 2003;79:1317–22.
33. Nastri CO, Lensen SF, Gibreel A, Raine-Fenning N, Ferriani RA, Bhattacharya S, et al. Endometrial injury in women undergoing assisted reproductive techniques. Cochrane Database Syst Rev. 2015;7:CD009517.
34. Coughlan C, Ledger W, Wang Q, Liu F, Demirol A, Gurgan T, et al. Recurrent implantation failure: definition and management. Reprod Biomed Online. 2014;28:14–38.
35. Aleyasin A, Abediasl Z, Nazari A, Sheikh M. Granulocyte colony-stimulating factor in repeated IVF failure, a randomized trial. Reproduction. 2016;151:637–42.
36. Navali N, Gassemzadeh A, Farzadi L, Abdollahi S, Nouri M, Hamdi K, et al. Intrauterine administration of hCG immediately after oocyte retrieval and the outcome of ICSI: a randomized controlled trial. Hum Reprod. 2016;31:2520–6.
37. Santamaria X, Cabanillas S, Cervello I, Arbona C, Raga F, Ferro J, et al. Autologous cell therapy with CD133+ bone marrow-derived stem cells for refractory Asherman's syndrome and endometrial atrophy: a pilot cohort study. Hum Reprod. 2016;31:1087–96.
38. Roque M, Lattes K, Serra S, Sola I, Geber S, Carreras R, et al. Fresh embryo transfer versus frozen embryo transfer in in vitro fertilization cycles: a systematic review and meta-analysis. Fertil Steril. 2013;99:156–62.
39. Berger S, Bleich M, Schmid W, Cole TJ, Peters J, Watanabe H, et al. Mineralocorticoid receptor knockout mice: pathophysiology of Na+ metabolism. Proc Natl Acad Sci U S A. 1998;95:9424–9.
40. Ng SC, Gilman-Sachs A, Thaker P, Beaman KD, Beer AE, Kwak-Kim J. Expression of intracellular Th1 and Th2 cytokines in women with recurrent spontaneous abortion, implantation failures after IVF/ET or normal pregnancy. Am J Reprod Immunol. 2002;48:77–86.
41. Nakagawa K, Kwak-Kim J, Ota K, Kuroda K, Hisano M, Sugiyama R, et al. Immunosuppression with tacrolimus improved reproductive outcome of women with repeated implantation failure and elevated peripheral blood Th1/Th2 cell ratios. Am J Reprod Immunol. 2015;73:353–61.

42. Nakagawa K, Kuroda K, Sugiyama R, Yamaguchi K. After 12 consecutive miscarriages, a patient received immunosuppressive treatment and delivered an intact baby. Reprod Med Biol. 2017;16:297–301.
43. Winger EE, Reed JL, Ashoush S, Ahuja S, El-Toukhy T, Taranissi M. Treatment with adalimumab (Humira((R))) and intravenous immunoglobulin improves pregnancy rates in women undergoing IVF. Am J Reprod Immunol. 2009;61:113–20.
44. Chambers CD, Johnson DL. Emerging data on the use of anti-tumor necrosis factor-alpha medications in pregnancy. Birth Defects Res A Clin Mol Teratol. 2012;94:607–11.
45. Ostensen M, Forger F. How safe are anti-rheumatic drugs during pregnancy? Curr Opin Pharmacol. 2013;13:470–5.
46. Brannstrom M, Johannesson L, Bokstrom H, Kvarnstrom N, Molne J, Dahm-Kahler P, et al. Livebirth after uterus transplantation. Lancet. 2015;385:607–16.
47. Tang AW, Alfirevic Z, Quenby S. Natural killer cells and pregnancy outcomes in women with recurrent miscarriage and infertility: a systematic review. Hum Reprod. 2011;26:1971–80.
48. Boomsma CM, Keay SD, Macklon NS. Peri-implantation glucocorticoid administration for assisted reproductive technology cycles. Cochrane Database Syst Rev. 2007;6:CD005996.
49. Mirzakhani H, Litonjua AA, McElrath TF, O'Connor G, Lee-Parritz A, Iverson R, et al. Early pregnancy vitamin D status and risk of preeclampsia. J Clin Invest. 2016;126:4702–15.
50. Rudick BJ, Ingles SA, Chung K, Stanczyk FZ, Paulson RJ, Bendikson KA. Influence of vitamin D levels on in vitro fertilization outcomes in donor-recipient cycles. Fertil Steril. 2014;101:447–52.
51. Fabris A, Pacheco A, Cruz M, Puente JM, Fatemi H, Garcia-Velasco JA. Impact of circulating levels of total and bioavailable serum vitamin D on pregnancy rate in egg donation recipients. Fertil Steril. 2014;102:1608–12.
52. Chiang N, Bermudez EA, Ridker PM, Hurwitz S, Serhan CN. Aspirin triggers antiinflammatory 15-epi-lipoxin A4 and inhibits thromboxane in a randomized human trial. Proc Natl Acad Sci U S A. 2004;101:15178–83.
53. Schisterman EF, Silver RM, Lesher LL, Faraggi D, Wactawski-Wende J, Townsend JM, et al. Preconception low-dose aspirin and pregnancy outcomes: results from the EAGeR randomised trial. Lancet. 2014;384:29–36.
54. Mumford SL, Silver RM, Sjaarda LA, Wactawski-Wende J, Townsend JM, Lynch AM, et al. Expanded findings from a randomized controlled trial of preconception low-dose aspirin and pregnancy loss. Hum Reprod. 2016;31:657–65.
55. Stern C, Chamley L, Norris H, Hale L, Baker HW. A randomized, double-blind, placebo-controlled trial of heparin and aspirin for women with in vitro fertilization implantation failure and antiphospholipid or antinuclear antibodies. Fertil Steril. 2003;80:376–83.
56. Colicchia M, Campagnolo L, Baldini E, Ulisse S, Valensise H, Moretti C. Molecular basis of thyrotropin and thyroid hormone action during implantation and early development. Hum Reprod Update. 2014;20:884–904.
57. Vissenberg R, Manders VD, Mastenbroek S, Fliers E, Afink GB, Ris-Stalpers C, et al. Pathophysiological aspects of thyroid hormone disorders/thyroid peroxidase autoantibodies and reproduction. Hum Reprod Update. 2015;21:378–87.

Part II
Unexplained Recurrent Miscarriage

Chapter 7
Unexplained Recurrent Miscarriage: Introduction

Keiji Kuroda

Abstract Recurrent miscarriage (RM) remains unexplained in >50% of patients and causes both physical and psychological burdens in women without specific risk factors for miscarriage. Unexplained RM is defined as a failure to achieve delivery owing to chance or undetectable causes of pregnancy loss, including unbalanced maternal immune tolerance, impaired intrauterine circumstances, and perturbation of decidualized endometrium. In 60–70% of patients with a history of three to four miscarriages, delivery is achieved without any treatment, whereas the miscarriage rate in patients with five or more pregnancy losses is >50%, of which ≥60% are losses of fetuses with normal embryonic karyotypes. Thus, the rate of miscarriage and the number of losses of fetuses with normal embryonic karyotype increase with an increase in the number of pregnancy losses, suggesting that maternal, not fetal, risk factors are present in patients with a history of multiple pregnancy losses. However, 75% of patients with unexplained RM achieve delivery after an appropriate treatment.

Keywords Unexplained recurrent miscarriage · Pregnancy loss · Decidualization

Recurrent pregnancy loss (RPL) is defined as the loss of two or more pregnancies, including biochemical pregnancy loss and pregnancy of unknown location. Recurrent miscarriage (RM) is defined as the loss of all pregnancies detected in the intrauterine cavity. In human beings, the incidence of embryo wastage is estimated to be 30% before implantation, 30% before 6 weeks of gestation (biochemical pregnancy loss), and 10–15% of clinical pregnancies (miscarriages, mainly before 12 weeks) [1]. Pregnancy loss is common in clinical practice; 38% of women with a history of pregnancy experience spontaneous abortion [2]. The accidental RM rate, but not the RPL rate, can be estimated as a common clinical miscarriage rate: 10–15% to the power of the number of miscarriages (n) or 0.1^n–0.15^n. Two and three

K. Kuroda
Center for Reproductive Medicine and Implantation Research, Sugiyama Clinic Shinjuku, Tokyo, Japan

Department of Obstetrics and Gynaecology, Faculty of Medicine, Juntendo University, Tokyo, Japan
e-mail: arthur@juntendo.ac.jp

© Springer Nature Singapore Pte Ltd. 2018
K. Kuroda et al. (eds.), *Treatment Strategy for Unexplained Infertility and Recurrent Miscarriage*, https://doi.org/10.1007/978-981-10-8690-8_7

Table 7.1 Recurrent miscarriage testing

- Interview for pregnancy history, lifestyle and health behavior
- Confirmation of anatomical uterine form and intrauterine cavity
  Ultrasonography, hysterosalpingography, pelvic MR imaging, hysteroscopy
- Metabolic and endocrinologic factors
  Ovarian and pituitary hormone (LH, FSH, prolactin, estradiol, progesterone)
  Thyroid hormone (free T3, free T4, TSH)
  Diabetes testing (blood sugar and insulin levels)
- Immunological investigation
  Antinuclear antibody, antiphospholipid antibody (lupus anticoagulant, anticardiolipin antibody: IgG, IgM, anti-β2-GP1 antibody: IgG, IgM, anti-phosphatidylethanolamine (PE) antibody: IgG, IgM)
  (Antithyroglobulin antibody, antiperoxidase antibody, TSH receptor antibody)
- Thrombophilia screening
  PT, APTT, protein C activity, protein S activity, factor XII
- Chromosomal testing for couple

consecutive miscarriages accidentally occur at rates of 1–3% and 0.1–0.3%, respectively, which are significantly lower frequencies than the true rates of 4.2% and 0.9%, respectively [2]. Women with a history of RPL experience both physical and psychological burdens. Therefore, patients with a history of RM require screening for the risk factors for miscarriage.

The components of RM assessment are shown in Table 7.1. Pregnancy loss is associated with a wide variety of risk factors. Interviewing patients about their pregnancy histories, lifestyle, and health behavior is particularly critical. Smoking, obesity, alcohol consumption, and caffeine intake are potential causes of pregnancy losses. Ultrasonography can be used to detect uterine malformation and organic diseases, including uterine myoma, and hysteroscopy can identify intrauterine disorders such as endometrial polyps and chronic endometritis. Blood analyses for RM include endocrinologic, immunological, and chromosomal tests and thrombophilia screening.

Overt thyroid disorder and thyroid autoimmunity are also involved in pregnancy loss [3, 4], whereas subclinical hypothyroidism and Hashimoto's disease (chronic thyroiditis) with normal thyroid hormone levels are associated with subfertility [4]. The detection of impaired thyroid hormone secretion signals a need to measure thyroid antibodies (for the diagnosis of Hashimoto's disease and Graves' disease), antithyroglobulin antibody, antiperoxidase antibody, and thyroid-stimulating hormone receptor antibody.

Although the association between polycystic ovary syndrome and pregnancy loss remains controversial, diagnosing polycystic ovary syndrome and examining patients for diabetes mellitus, including insulin resistance, are critical. Immunological investigations mainly test for antiphospholipid antibody syndrome and include the following three antibodies: lupus anticoagulant, anticardiolipin antibody, and anti-β2-GP1 antibody. The presence of anti-phosphatidylethanolamine antibody

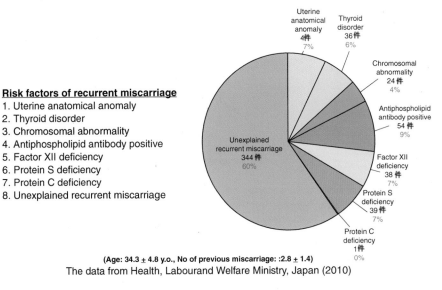

Risk factors of recurrent miscarriage
1. Uterine anatomical anomaly
2. Thyroid disorder
3. Chromosomal abnormality
4. Antiphospholipid antibody positive
5. Factor XII deficiency
6. Protein S deficiency
7. Protein C deficiency
8. Unexplained recurrent miscarriage

(Age: 34.3 ± 4.8 y.o., No of previous miscarriage: :2.8 ± 1.4)
The data from Health, Labourand Welfare Ministry, Japan (2010)

Fig. 7.1 Frequency of risk factors for recurrent miscarriage. Risk factors for recurrent miscarriage include uterine anatomical anomalies, thyroid disorders, chromosomal abnormalities, antiphospholipid antibody syndrome, factor XII deficiency, and protein S and C deficiency. Data from the Health, Labour and Welfare Ministry of Japan show that more than half of RMs are owing to unexplained risk factors. The data from Health, Labour and Welfare Ministry, Japan (2010) (http://fuiku.jp/study/)

should also be tested. Measurements of protein C and S and factor XII activity are also required during thrombophilia screening.

A research group at the Health, Labour and Welfare Ministry of Japan investigated the frequency of risk factors for RM (http://fuiku.jp/study/) and found rates of approximately 25% for thrombophilia, including antiphospholipid antibody syndrome, 7.8% for organic factors such as uterine malformation, 6.8% for thyroid disorder, and >50% for unexplained factors (Fig. 7.1). If the presence of antiphosphatidylethanolamine antibody is included among the risk factors for pregnancy loss, approximately 40% of patients with RM have no risk factors. Other reports have also shown that unexplained RM occurs in a high proportion of the population [5].

Patients with unexplained RM include those who do not achieve delivery owing to chance or undetectable causes of pregnancy loss. Given the association between the number of previous miscarriages and the miscarriage rate for the next pregnancy, 60–70% of patients with a history of three to four miscarriages eventually achieve delivery without treatment, whereas the miscarriage rate in patients with five or more pregnancy losses is >50%, of which ≥60% are losses of fetuses with normal embryonic karyotype [6]. Thus, the rate of miscarriage and the number of

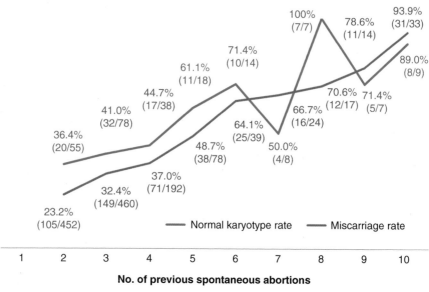

Ogasawara M, Fertil Steril, 2000

Fig. 7.2 Miscarriage rates and normal embryonic karyotype rates. The figure shows the association between the number of previous miscarriages and the miscarriage rates and the rates of normal embryonic karyotype in subsequent pregnancies. The rates of miscarriage and normal embryonic karyotype increase with an increase in the number of pregnancy losses. Ogasawara, Fertil Steril, 2000

losses of fetuses with a normal embryonic karyotype increase with the increase in the number of pregnancy losses, suggesting that maternal, not fetal, risk factors are present in patients with a history of RPL (Fig. 7.2) [6]. Candidate risk factors in unexplained RM include unbalanced maternal immune tolerance for the maintenance of pregnancy, impaired intrauterine circumstances at the local implantation site, and perturbation of the decidualization of uterine endometrium.

Recent studies suggest that decidualized endometrial stromal cells serve as biosensors of embryo quality at implantation [7–10]. Unexplained RM is associated with an aberrantly high number of uterine natural killer cells and the abnormal proliferation of angiogenesis in the local uterine endometrium, which indicate a highly receptive environment for embryos [1, 7, 8, 11]. More than half of the pregnancy losses in patients with RM having no specific risk factors are related to embryonic chromosomal anomalies [5]. Unexplained RM may be partial because of inadequate endometrial receptivity of the decidualized endometrium to preimplantation embryos that should have been wasted (natural embryo selection hypothesis), whereas poor endometrial receptivity and excessive embryo selection of the uterine endometrium may result in recurrent implantation failure (Fig. 7.3) [10, 12].

Most women with a history of RM become anxious during their subsequent pregnancies [13], and maternal stress is associated with an increased risk of preg-

Fig. 7.3 Natural embryo selection hypothesis. There is a balance between selective and receptive functions of the decidualized endometrium. Decidualized endometrium with high receptivity may result in miscarriage with an aneuploid embryo, whereas high selectivity is associated with implantation failure, even with euploid embryos. Gellersen, Brosen, Endocr Rev. 2014

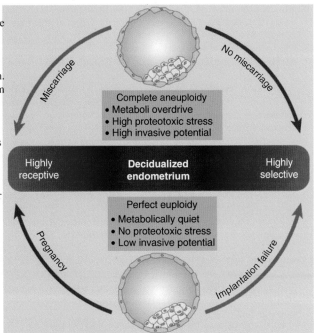

Gellersen B and Brosen JJ, Endocr Rev. 2014

nancy loss [14]. The lack of specific risk factors for miscarriage is a source of further anxiety in patients with RM, leading to a vicious cycle of pregnancy loss. However, 75% of patients with unexplained RM can maintain pregnancies to delivery after proper evaluation and treatment [15, 16]. This book aimed to improve the understanding of unexplained RM and help caregivers reduce stress in patients with RM by offering data regarding the high likelihood of eventual delivery through appropriate treatments.

References

1. Teklenburg G, Salker M, Heijnen C, Macklon NS, Brosens JJ. The molecular basis of recurrent pregnancy loss: impaired natural embryo selection. Mol Hum Reprod. 2010;16:886–95.
2. Sugiura-Ogasawara M, Suzuki S, Ozaki Y, Katano K, Suzumori N, Kitaori T. Frequency of recurrent spontaneous abortion and its influence on further marital relationship and illness: the Okazaki Cohort Study in Japan. J Obstet Gynaecol Res. 2013;39:126–31.
3. Vissenberg R, Manders VD, Mastenbroek S, Fliers E, Afink GB, Ris-Stalpers C, Goddijn M, Bisschop PH. Pathophysiological aspects of thyroid hormone disorders/thyroid peroxidase autoantibodies and reproduction. Hum Reprod Update. 2015;21:378–87.
4. De Groot L, Abalovich M, Alexander EK, Amino N, Barbour L, Cobin RH, Eastman CJ, Lazarus JH, Luton D, Mandel SJ, Mestman J, Rovet J, Sullivan S. Management of thyroid dysfunction during pregnancy and postpartum: an endocrine society clinical practice guideline. J Clin Endocrinol Metab. 2012;97:2543–65.

5. Sugiura-Ogasawara M, Ozaki Y, Katano K, Suzumori N, Kitaori T, Mizutani E. Abnormal embryonic karyotype is the most frequent cause of recurrent miscarriage. Hum Reprod. 2012;27:2297–303.

6. Ogasawara M, Aoki K, Okada S, Suzumori K. Embryonic karyotype of abortuses in relation to the number of previous miscarriages. Fertil Steril. 2000;73:300–4.

7. Teklenburg G, Salker M, Molokhia M, Lavery S, Trew G, Aojanepong T, Mardon HJ, Lokugamage AU, Rai R, Landles C, Roelen BAJ, Quenby S, Kuijk EW, Kavelaars A, Heijnen CJ, Regan L, Brosens JJ, Macklon NS. Natural selection of human embryos: decidualizing endometrial stromal cells serve as sensors of embryo quality upon implantation. PLoS One. 2010;5:e10258.

8. Weimar CHE, Kavelaars A, Brosens JJ, Gellersen B, de Vreeden-Elbertse JMT, Heijnen CJ, Macklon NS. Endometrial stromal cells of women with recurrent miscarriage fail to discriminate between high-and low-quality human embryos. PLoS One. 2012;7:e41424.

9. Brosens JJ, Salker MS, Teklenburg G, Nautiyal J, Salter S, Lucas ES, Steel JH, Christian M, Chan Y-W, Boomsma CM, Moore JD, Hartshorne GM, Sucurovic S, Mulac-Jericevic B, Heijnen CJ, Quenby S, Koerkamp MJG, Holstege FCP, Shmygol A, Macklon NS. Uterine selection of human embryos at implantation. Sci Rep. 2014;4:3894.

10. Macklon NS, Brosens JJ. The human endometrium as a sensor of embryo quality. Biol Reprod. 2014;91:98.

11. Salker M, Teklenburg G, Molokhia M, Lavery S, Trew G, Aojanepong T, Mardon HJ, Lokugamage AU, Rai R, Landles C, Roelen BAJ, Quenby S, Kuijk EW, Kavelaars A, Heijnen CJ, Regan L, Macklon NS, Brosens JJ. Natural selection of human embryos: impaired decidualization of endometrium disables embryo-maternal interactions and causes recurrent pregnancy loss. PLoS One. 2010;5:e10287.

12. Gellersen B, Brosens JJ. Cyclic Decidualization of the human endometrium in reproductive health and failure. Endocr Rev. 2014;35:851–905.

13. Kolte AM, Olsen LR, Mikkelsen EM, Christiansen OB, Nielsen HS. Depression and emotional stress is highly prevalent among women with recurrent pregnancy loss. Hum Reprod. 2015;30:777–82.

14. Li W, Newell-Price J, Jones GL, Ledger WL, Li TC. Relationship between psychological stress and recurrent miscarriage. Reprod Biomed Online. 2012;25:180–9.

15. Clifford K, Rai R, Regan L. Future pregnancy outcome in unexplained recurrent first trimester miscarriage. Hum Reprod. 1997;12:387–9.

16. Brigham SA, Conlon C, Farquharson RG. A longitudinal study of pregnancy outcome following idiopathic recurrent miscarriage. Hum Reprod. 1999;14:2868–71.

Chapter 8
Previous Trial Studies of Unexplained Recurrent Miscarriage

Keiji Kuroda

Abstract Women with unexplained recurrent miscarriage (RM) cannot achieve a live birth because of accidental sporadic repeated miscarriages or miscarriages due to undetectable causes. Previous trial studies of unexplained RM treatment include the use of low-dose aspirin, low-molecular-weight heparin, lymphocyte immunization therapy, intravenous immunoglobulin (IVIG), prednisolone, and progesterone. Currently, there is no established treatment for unexplained RM. The use of preconception IVIG or the systemic administration of dydrogesterone is a promising treatment for the prevention of pregnancy loss. And postconception prednisolone treatment may also be an efficacy for RM patients with elevated uNK cells. Yet the evidence is still insufficient. The optimization of maternal immune tolerance and decidualization of the endometrium may be crucial therapies for unexplained RM.

Keywords Unexplained recurrent miscarriage · Low-dose aspirin · Low-molecular-weight heparin · Lymphocyte immunization therapy · Intravenous immunoglobulin · Prednisolone · Progesterone

8.1 Introduction

Given the association between the number of previous miscarriages and the miscarriage rate for subsequent pregnancies, 60–70% of patients with a history of three to four miscarriages eventually achieve delivery without treatment. However, the miscarriage rate in patients with five or more pregnancy losses is >50%, of which ≥60% are fetus losses with a normal karyotype of the conception products [1]. Therefore, the miscarriage and normal embryonic karyotype rates increase with the rise in the number of

---

K. Kuroda
Center for Reproductive Medicine and Implantation Research, Sugiyama Clinic Shinjuku, Tokyo, Japan

Department of Obstetrics and Gynaecology, Faculty of Medicine, Juntendo University, Tokyo, Japan
e-mail: arthur@juntendo.ac.jp

© Springer Nature Singapore Pte Ltd. 2018
K. Kuroda et al. (eds.), *Treatment Strategy for Unexplained Infertility and Recurrent Miscarriage*, https://doi.org/10.1007/978-981-10-8690-8_8

pregnancy losses, suggesting that maternal, not fetal, risk factors are present in patients with a history of five or more miscarriages [1]. Established risk factors for recurrent miscarriage (RM) include thrombophilia (e.g., antiphospholipid syndrome), uterine malformation, parental chromosomal abnormalities, and thyroid disorder [2–4]. According to previous reports, unexplained RM occurs in approximately half of women with a history of RM [2, 5–7]. Women with unexplained RM may not achieve live birth due to accidental sporadic repeated pregnancy losses. Gynecologists, however, should provide therapy to the patients suffering from RM because they presumptively have an undetectable cause of pregnancy loss. Candidate risk factors in unexplained RM include unknown thrombophilia, unbalanced maternal immune tolerance, perturbed intrauterine circumstances, and impaired decidualization of the uterine endometrium. A large number of trial studies for unexplained RM have been performed.

8.2 Anticoagulants

8.2.1 Low-Dose Aspirin (LDA)

Thrombophilic disorder is one of the most popular causes of RM. Extensively studied, the use of LDA for RM has been established as the postconception treatment for the prevention of miscarriage in women with thrombophilia factors [8, 9]. Schisterman et al. compared the results of live birth rates between women with LDA treatment and placebo (EAGeR randomized trial) [10]. Of 1078 women with a history of one-to-two spontaneous pregnancy losses, 535 given preconception-initiated daily LDA (81 mg/day) and folic acid treatment were compared with 543 given placebo and folic acid supplementation for up to six menstrual cycles. The treatment continued postconception, until 36 weeks of gestation. The live birth rates in the LDA and placebo groups were 57.8% (309 of 535 women) and 52.7% (286 of 543 women), respectively [relative risk (RR) = 1.10, 95% confidence interval (CI) -0.84–11.02; $p = 0.098$]. Miscarriage rates were 12.7% (68 women) and 12.0% (65 women), respectively (RR = 1.06, 95% CI 0.77–1.46; $p = 0.78$). Therefore, LDA treatment cannot prevent miscarriage in women with repeated pregnancy losses.

8.2.2 Low-Molecular-Weight Heparin (LMWH)

Previous studies have shown that LMWH increases the live birth rate in pregnant women with known thrombophilia [11, 12]. Schleussner et al. assessed whether LMWH increases live birth rates in women with unexplained RM [13]. Of 440 women with a history of a minimum of two consecutive early miscarriages or one late miscarriage, 220 women, who received multivitamin supplementation and 5000 IU of dalteparin sodium for up to 24 weeks' gestation, were compared with 214 women receiving multivitamin supplementation (control group). At 24 weeks gestation, ongoing pregnancy rates in the intervention and control groups were 86.8% (191 of 220 pregnancies) and 87.9% (188 of 214 pregnancies), respectively (95% CI −7.4–5.3; $p = 0.75$). The live birth rates were 86.0% and 86.7%, respectively (95% CI −7.3–5.9; $p = 0.84$). The use of LMWH does not contribute to an increase in ongoing pregnancy and live birth rates in women with unexplained RM. A meta-analysis of prospective, randomized trials for the use of LMWH in women with unexplained RM did not confirm this benefit [14]. There is an additional risk of heparin-induced thrombocytopenia and osteoporosis [15]. Thus, LMWH injections for unexplained RM are not recommended.

8.3 Immunological Regulator

8.3.1 The Effect of Maternal Immunity on Pregnancy Loss

Maternal immune tolerance, involved in natural killer (NK) and helper T cells, plays a vital role in the establishment of a successful pregnancy by facilitating the immunologic adaptation of the semi-allogenic developing embryo. The impact of maternal immunity on miscarriage is summarized in Table 8.1. Aoki et al. reported that elevated preconceptional peripheral blood NK (pNK) cell activity may be predictive of subsequent miscarriage in 68 patients with two consecutive pregnancy losses [16]. Miscarriage rates in the women with aberrant elevated and normal pNK cell activities were 71% (17 of 24 women) and 20% (9 of 44 women), respectively (RR = 3.5, 95% CI 1.8–6.5). Later trials, however, demonstrated no differences in pNK cell activities between the patients with RM and controls [17–19].

CD56^{bright} and CD16$^-$ uterine NK (uNK) cells are entirely different from circulating pNK cells (CD56^{dim} and CD16$^+$) [20, 21]. uNK cells, which have little cytotoxic activity, are thought to play a significant role in the establishment and maintenance of early pregnancy via endometrial angiogenesis, remodeling of uterine spiral arteries, and trophoblast invasion, which are essential for a normal pregnancy [22]. Several articles have reported a relationship between unexplained RM and aberrant high uNK cell density in mid-luteal phase endometrial cells [23–25]. Quenby et al. proposed that uNK cells increase endometrial vessel formation, thereby increasing

Table 8.1 Candidate risk factors of recurrent miscarriage in immunological regulators

Immune cells	Relationship with recurrent miscarriage	References
Peripheral NK cell (CD56^{dim} and CD16$^+$)	No relationship	Emmer et al. [17] Souza et al. [18] Wang et al. [19]
Uterine NK cell (CD56^{bright} and CD16$^-$)	Controversial (insufficient evidence)	Quenby et al. [23]
Helper T cell	Controversial (insufficient evidence)	Lee et al. [28] Makhseed et al. [29]

uterine artery blood flow, leading to excessive oxidative stress in the early placenta [23]. Yet the evidence is still insufficient.

The maternal immune system for pregnancy is involved in balancing T-helper (Th) cells, including Th1 cells [interleukin (IL)-2, tumor necrosis factor (TNF)-α, and interferon-γ production] and Th2 cells (IL-4, IL-5, and IL-10 production), in favor of Th2 cells [26, 27]. An impaired Th-cell population may result in reproductive failure, including infertility and miscarriage. In peripheral blood lymphocytes, the level of Th1 cells expressing TNF-α in women with RM was found to be higher than that in fertile women [28]. Additionally, the level of Th2 cytokines in women with RM who ended in miscarriage was significantly lower than that in fertile pregnant women and women with RM who completed live birth [29]. However, the relationship between aberrant Th1/Th2 cell balance and RM is still controversial.

8.3.2 Lymphocyte Immunization Therapy (LIT)

In a randomized controlled trial, Mowbray et al. reported a beneficial effect of allogeneic LIT in women with RM [30]. It is known that LIT can produce anti-paternal antibodies or defensive antibodies from fetus rejection that are lacking in women with a history of RM [31]. A systematic review based on 12 randomized controlled trials has shown an odds ratio (OR) for live birth in patients with LIT using paternal lymphocytes of 1.23 (95% CI 0.89–1.70). Further, three trials using third-party lymphocytes have demonstrated an OR of 1.39 (95% CI 0.68–2.82); thus, there was no significant effect of LIT treatment on the live birth rates in patients with RM [32]. Treatment with allogeneic cells raises severe risks, including exposure to blood-borne viruses, neonatal alloimmune thrombocytopenia, and the production of red blood cell antibodies, leading to erythroblastosis fetalis [33]. Therefore, LIT should not be used as a treatment for unexplained RM.

8.3.3 Intravenous Immunoglobulin (IVIG)

In the late 1980s, passive immunization with IVIG was reported to have beneficial effects as a treatment for RM [34]. The underlying mechanism may be associated with the neutralization of autoantibodies in the circulatory system, inhibition of NK cells, attenuation of complement-mediated cytotoxicity, and release of regulatory T lymphocytes [35]. Clinically, IVIG has been widely used to treat unexplained RM, although its efficacy has not yet been clinically proven [36]. The high cost, limited supply, and potential side effects of this immunotherapy call for a guideline for appropriate application. Wang et al. reported the currently available randomized controlled trials to determine the effectiveness of IVIG in improving the chance of live birth in patients with unexplained RM [37]. The 11 included studies were high-quality trials with a low risk of babies. In total, 582 patients achieved pregnancy; 297 patients were in the IVIG treatment group for RM, and 285 patients were in the placebo group. A total of 202 (68.0%) and 151 (53.0%) live births occurred in the IVIG and placebo groups, respectively (RR = 1.25, 95% CI 1.00–1.56; p = 0.05). This random-effects analysis showed that the difference in the live birth rates between IVIG treatment and placebo groups was on the margin of significance.

The effect of IVIG on the live birth rate, when administered before or after conception, was also analyzed. In total, 213 women who had experienced RM and initiated treatment with either IVIG or placebo before the confirmation of pregnancy and 369 women who had experienced RM and were treated with IVIG or placebo after conception were evaluated. In the preconception group, 80 of 107 women (74.8%) treated with IVIG and 47 of 106 women (44.3%) treated with placebo achieved a live birth (RR = 1.67, 95% CI 1.30–2.14; p < 0.05), whereas in the post-conception group, 122 of 190 women (64.2%) treated with IVIG and 104 of 179 women (58.1%) treated with placebo achieved a live birth (RR = 1.10, 95% CI 0.93–1.29; p = 0.27). These data suggest that women with unexplained RM may benefit from IVIG administered before conception. However, the evidence is not sufficient to prove the beneficial effects of IVIG in patients with unexplained RM. Further studies are required to elucidate the effectiveness of IVIG.

8.3.4   Prednisolone

Glucocorticoids, such as prednisolone, can suppress excess numbers of uNK cells and abnormal angiogenesis in the endometrium [25, 38, 39]. Therefore, successful live births in patients with RM with abnormally high levels of uNK cells after prednisolone treatment have been reported [38]. In a randomized controlled trial, Tang et al. [40] demonstrated the impact of prednisolone treatment (20 mg for 6 weeks, 10 mg for 1 week, and 5 mg for 1 week) in women with RM who had a high density of uNK cells. The live birth rate in the prednisolone group was higher (60.0%; 12 of 20 women) than that in the placebo group (40.0%; 8 of 20 women) (RR = 1.5, 95% CI 0.8–2.9), yet there was no significant difference. In this study, the number of entry patients with RM was low; thus, further prednisolone trials are warranted. Regarding implantation, an inflammatory response with proinflammatory cytokines and prostaglandins is an essential process for the embryo to attach and invade the decidual endometrium [41–43]. As a precaution for the use of prednisolone for the prevention of miscarriage, administration after implantation is recommended.

8.4   Optimization of Decidualization of Endometrium

8.4.1   Progesterone

Progesterone is an indispensable hormone for decidualization of the endometrium, implantation, and maintenance of pregnancy. Progesterone is also an activator of local cortisone during the decidual transformation of the endometrium, leading to the direct and indirect regulation of uNK cell density via glucocorticoid receptors [25, 44, 45]. Progesterone can further inhibit the contraction of uterine smooth muscles and the production of prostaglandins and induce the production of Th2 cell cytokines, leading to the optimization of immune tolerance for an embryo [46]. Therefore, progesterone is expected to be therapeutically efficacious for RM via modulation of maternal immune tolerance as well as decidualization of uterine endometrium. A systematic review including four small trials has demonstrated that the miscarriage rate in women receiving progesterone treatment is significantly lower than that in women receiving placebo or no treatment (OR = 0.39, 95% CI 0.21–0.72) [47]. Coomarasamy et al. [48] reported a multicenter, randomized controlled trial (PROMISE study) of vaginal progesterone suppositories (400 mg twice daily) for women with unexplained RM. Of 836 women with three or more prior miscarriages, the live birth rate in the progesterone group was 65.8% (262 of 398 women), which was comparable to the 63.3% (271 of 428 women) rate in the placebo group (RR = 1.04, 95% CI 0.94–1.15; $p = 0.45$). Thus, a vaginal progesterone suppository is not beneficial as a treatment for unexplained RM.

Conversely, according to a systematic review [49, 50], it has been revealed that synthetic progestogen, including dydrogesterone, has a therapeutic effect on unexplained RM. In particular, Kumar et al. [51] demonstrated the impact of dydrogesterone treatment (10 mg twice daily) on unexplained RM via the regulation of Th cell cytokines. Therefore, the systemic administration of synthetic progestogen may be a beneficial treatment for women with RM, compared with vaginal natural progesterone treatment. Significantly, progesterone treatment has no harmful effects on implantation, placentation, and the fetus.

8.5   Past and Future Trials for Unexplained RM

Previous trial studies for unexplained RM are summarized in Table 8.2. The data demonstrate that there is no established treatment for unexplained RM. A highlight in previous trials is high live birth rates in the placebo groups. Thus there had been no significant difference, but some treatments are to be used as placebo for "tender loving care," psychological support. The use of preconception IVIG or the systemic administration of dydrogesterone is a promising treatment, but the evidence is still insufficient. These treatments can modulate maternal immune tolerance, including balancing Th cells and the decidualization of the endometrium. And postconception prednisolone treatment may also be an efficacy for selecting RM patients with elevated uNK cells. Although the relationship between RM and inappropriate maternal Th cell levels is still debatable, notable treatment for unexplained RM includes immunosuppressive drugs, such as tacrolimus and cyclosporine, for the regulation of the Th1/Th2 cell ratio [52, 53]. Vitamin D also modulates Th cells in several organ systems, and vitamin D deficiency is associated with many autoimmune diseases [54]. Unexplained RM is also linked to the lack of maternal vitamin D [55].

Table 8.2 Past trial studies for unexplained recurrent miscarriage

Treatment	Recommendation	Comments	References
Low-dose aspirin (LDA)	No recommendation	LDA should not be administered before implantation	Schisterman et al. [10]
Low-molecular-weight heparin (LMWH)	No recommendation	There is a risk of heparin-induced thrombocytopenia	Schleussner et al. [13]
Lymphocyte immunization therapy	No recommendation	There is a risk of neonatal alloimmune thrombocytopenia and production of red blood cell antibodies	Wong et al. [32]
Intravenous immunoglobulin (IVIG)	IVIG treatment before conception may improve live birth rate	IVIG should be administered before conception Very expensive, thus the period of treatment is limited	Wang et al. [37]
Prednisolone	Prednisolone may improve live birth rate in women with high uterine NK cell level, but the number of trials is insufficient	Prednisolone should not be administered before implantation	Tang et al. [40]
Progesterone	Dydrogesterone may improve live birth rate, but the evidence is still insufficient	No adverse effect	Coomarasamy et al. [48] Kumar et al. [51]

These approaches, with the use or combination of dydrogesterone, prednisolone, vitamin D, and immunosuppressive drugs, may prove to be an effective future therapy for unexplained RM.

References

1. Ogasawara M, Aoki K, Okada S, Suzumori K. Embryonic karyotype of abortuses in relation to the number of previous miscarriages. Fertil Steril. 2000;73:300–4.
2. Sugiura-Ogasawara M, Ozaki Y, Katano K, Suzumori N, Kitaori T, Mizutani E. Abnormal embryonic karyotype is the most frequent cause of recurrent miscarriage. Hum Reprod. 2012;27:2297–303.
3. Branch DW, Gibson M, Silver RM. Clinical practice. Recurrent miscarriage. N Engl J Med. 2010;363:1740–7.
4. Farquharson RG, Pearson JF, John L. Lupus anticoagulant and pregnancy management. Lancet. 1984;2:228–9.
5. Clifford K, Rai R, Watson H, Regan L. An informative protocol for the investigation of recurrent miscarriage: preliminary experience of 500 consecutive cases. Hum Reprod. 1994;9:1328–32.
6. Stephenson MD. Frequency of factors associated with habitual abortion in 197 couples. Fertil Steril. 1996;66:24–9.
7. Jaslow CR, Carney JL, Kutteh WH. Diagnostic factors identified in 1020 women with two versus three or more recurrent pregnancy losses. Fertil Steril. 2010;93:1234–43.

8. Kaandorp S, Di Nisio M, Goddijn M, Middeldorp S. Aspirin or anticoagulants for treating recurrent miscarriage in women without antiphospholipid syndrome. Cochrane Database Syst Rev. 2009;1:Cd004734.

9. Kaandorp SP, Goddijn M, van der Post JA, Hutten BA, Verhoeve HR, Hamulyak K, Mol BW, Folkeringa N, Nahuis M, Papatsonis DN, Buller HR, van der Veen F, Middeldorp S. Aspirin plus heparin or aspirin alone in women with recurrent miscarriage. N Engl J Med. 2010;362:1586–96.

10. Schisterman EF, Silver RM, Lesher LL, Faraggi D, Wactawski-Wende J, Townsend JM, Lynch AM, Perkins NJ, Mumford SL, Galai N. Preconception low-dose aspirin and pregnancy outcomes: results from the EAGeR randomised trial. Lancet. 2014;384:29–36.

11. Brenner B, Hoffman R, Blumenfeld Z, Weiner Z, Younis JS. Gestational outcome in thrombophilic women with recurrent pregnancy loss treated by enoxaparin. Thromb Haemost. 2000;83:693–7.

12. Carp H, Dolitzky M, Inbal A. Thromboprophylaxis improves the live birth rate in women with consecutive recurrent miscarriages and hereditary thrombophilia. J Thromb Haemost. 2003;1:433–8.

13. Schleussner E, Kamin G, Seliger G, Rogenhofer N, Ebner S, Toth B, Schenk M, Henes M, Bohlmann MK, Fischer T, Brosteanu O, Bauersachs R, Petroff D, Grp E. Low-molecular-weight heparin for women with unexplained recurrent pregnancy loss a multicenter trial with a minimization randomization scheme. Ann Intern Med. 2015;162:601–U193.

14. Mantha S, Bauer KA, Zwicker JI. Low molecular weight heparin to achieve live birth following unexplained pregnancy loss: a systematic review. J Thromb Haemost. 2010;8:263–8.

15. Eldor A. The use of low-molecular-weight heparin for the management of venous thromboembolism in pregnancy. Eur J Obstet Gynecol Reprod Biol. 2002;104:3–13.

16. Aoki K, Kajiura S, Matsumoto Y, Ogasawara M, Okada S, Yagami Y, Gleicher N. Preconceptional natural-killer-cell activity as a predictor of miscarriage. Lancet. 1995;345:1340–2.

17. Emmer PM, Nelen WL, Steegers EA, Hendriks JC, Veerhoek M, Joosten I. Peripheral natural killer cytotoxity and CD56(pos)CD16(pos) cells increase during early pregnancy in women with a history of recurrent spontaneous abortion. Hum Reprod. 2000;15:1163–9.

18. Souza SS, Ferriani RA, Santos CM, Voltarelli JC. Immunological evaluation of patients with recurrent abortion. J Reprod Immunol. 2002;56:111–21.

19. Wang Q, Li TC, Wu YP, Cocksedge KA, Fu YS, Kong QY, Yao SZ. Reappraisal of peripheral NK cells in women with recurrent miscarriage. Reprod Biomed Online. 2008;17:814–9.

20. King A, Balendran N, Wooding P, Carter NP, Loke YW. CD3-leukocytes present in the human uterus during early placentation: phenotypic and morphologic characterization of the CD56++ population. Dev Immunol. 1991;1:169–90.

21. Nagler A, Lanier LL, Cwirla S, Phillips JH. Comparative studies of human FcRIII-positive and negative natural killer cells. J Immunol. 1989;143:3183–91.

22. Hanna J, Goldman-Wohl D, Hamani Y, Avraham I, Greenfield C, Natanson-Yaron S, Prus D, Cohen-Daniel L, Arnon TI, Manaster I, Gazit R, Yutkin V, Benharroch D, Porgador A, Keshet E, Yagel S, Mandelboim O. Decidual NK cells regulate key developmental processes at the human fetal-maternal interface. Nat Med. 2006;12:1065–74.

23. Quenby S, Nik H, Innes B, Lash G, Turner M, Drury J, Bulmer J. Uterine natural killer cells and angiogenesis in recurrent reproductive failure. Hum Reprod. 2009;24:45–54.

24. Clifford K, Flanagan AM, Regan L. Endometrial CD56+natural killer cells in women with recurrent miscarriage: a histomorphometric study. Hum Reprod. 1999;14:2727–30.

25. Kuroda K, Venkatakrishnan R, James S, Sucurovic S, Mulac-Jericevic B, Lucas ES, Takeda S, Shmygol A, Brosens JJ, Quenby S. Elevated periimplantation uterine natural killer cell density in human endometrium is associated with impaired corticosteroid signaling in decidualizing stromal cells. J Clin Endocrinol Metab. 2013;98:4429–37.

26. Raghupathy R, Makhseed M, Azizieh F, Omu A, Gupta M, Farhat R. Cytokine production by maternal lymphocytes during normal human pregnancy and in unexplained recurrent spontaneous abortion. Hum Reprod. 2000;15:713–8.

27. Ng SC, Gilman-Sachs A, Thaker P, Beaman KD, Beer AE, Kwak-Kim J. Expression of intracellular Th1 and Th2 cytokines in women with recurrent spontaneous abortion, implantation failures after IVF/ET or normal pregnancy. Am J Reprod Immunol. 2002;48:77–86.
28. Lee SK, Na BJ, Kim JY, Hur SE, Lee M, Gilman-Sachs A, Kwak-Kim J. Determination of clinical cellular immune markers in women with recurrent pregnancy loss. Am J Reprod Immunol. 2013;70:398–411.
29. Makhseed M, Raghupathy R, Azizieh F, Omu A, Al-Shamali E, Ashkanani L. Th1 and Th2 cytokine profiles in recurrent aborters with successful pregnancy and with subsequent abortions. Hum Reprod. 2001;16:2219–26.
30. Mowbray JF, Gibbings C, Liddell H, Reginald PW, Underwood JL, Beard RW. Controlled trial of treatment of recurrent spontaneous abortion by immunisation with paternal cells. Lancet. 1985;1:941–3.
31. Beer AE, Quebbeman JF, Ayers JW, Haines RF. Major histocompatibility complex antigens, maternal and paternal immune responses, and chronic habitual abortions in humans. Am J Obstet Gynecol. 1981;141:987–99.
32. Wong LF, Porter TF, Scott JR. Immunotherapy for recurrent miscarriage. Cochrane Database Syst Rev. 2014;2:CD000112.
33. Tanaka T, Umesaki N, Nishio J, Maeda K, Kawamura T, Araki N, Ogita S. Neonatal thrombocytopenia induced by maternal anti-HLA antibodies: a potential side effect of allogenic leukocyte immunization for unexplained recurrent aborters. J Reprod Immunol. 2000;46:51–7.
34. Mueller-Eckhardt G, Heine O, Neppert J, Kunzel W, Mueller-Eckhardt C. Prevention of recurrent spontaneous abortion by intravenous immunoglobulin. Vox Sang. 1989;56:151–4.
35. Schwab I, Nimmerjahn F. Intravenous immunoglobulin therapy: how does IgG modulate the immune system? Nat Rev Immunol. 2013;13:176–89.
36. Hutton L, Sharma R, Fergusson D, Tinmouth A, Hebert P, Jamieson J, Walker M. Use of intravenous immunoglobulin for treatment of recurrent miscarriage: a systematic review. BJOG. 2007;114:134–42.
37. Wang SW, Zhong SY, Lou LJ, Hu ZF, Sun HY, Zhu HY. The effect of intravenous immunoglobulin passive immunotherapy on unexplained recurrent spontaneous abortion: a meta-analysis. Reprod Biomed Online. 2016;33:720–36.
38. Quenby S, Kalumbi C, Bates M, Farquharson R, Vince G. Prednisolone reduces preconceptual endometrial natural killer cells in women with recurrent miscarriage. Fertil Steril. 2005;84:980–4.
39. Lash GE, Bulmer JN, Innes BA, Drury JA, Robson SC, Quenby S. Prednisolone treatment reduces endometrial spiral artery development in women with recurrent miscarriage. Angiogenesis. 2011;14:523–32.
40. Tang AW, Alfirevic Z, Turner MA, Drury J, Topping J, Dawood F, Farquharson R, Quenby S. A pilot, double blind randomised controlled trial of prednisolone for women with recurrent miscarriage and raised uterine natural killer cell density. Hum Reprod. 2011;26:268–1161.
41. Chard T. Cytokines in implantation. Hum Reprod Update. 1995;1:385–96.
42. Sharkey A. Cytokines and implantation. Rev Reprod. 1998;3:52–61.
43. Kelly RW, King AE, Critchley HOD. Cytokine control in human endometrium. Reproduction. 2001;121:3–19.
44. Kuroda K, Venkatakrishnan R, Salker MS, Lucas ES, Shaheen F, Kuroda M, Blanks A, Christian M, Quenby S, Brosens JJ. Induction of 11 beta-HSD 1 and activation of distinct mineralocorticoid receptor- and glucocorticoid receptor-dependent gene networks in decidualizing human endometrial stromal cells. Mol Endocrinol. 2013;27:192–202.
45. Guo W, Li PF, Zhao GF, Fan HY, Hu YL, Hou YY. Glucocorticoid receptor mediates the effect of progesterone on uterine natural killer cells. Am J Reprod Immunol. 2012;67:463–73.
46. Szekeres-Bartho J, Balasch J. Progestagen therapy for recurrent miscarriage. Hum Reprod Update. 2008;14:27–35.
47. Haas DM, Ramsey PS. Progestogen for preventing miscarriage. Cochrane Database Syst Rev. 2013;10:Cd003511.

48. Coomarasamy A, Williams H, Truchanowicz E, Seed PT, Small R, Quenby S, Gupta P, Dawood F, Koot YEM, Atik RB, Bloemenkamp KWM, Brady R, Briley AL, Cavallaro R, Cheong YC, Chu JJ, Eapen A, Ewies A, Hoek A, Kaaijk EM, Koks CAM, Li TC, MacLean M, Mol BW, Moore J, Ross JA, Sharpe L, Stewart J, Vaithilingam N, Farquharson RG, Kilby MD, Khalaf Y, Goddijn M, Regan L, Rai R. A randomized trial of progesterone in women with recurrent miscarriages. N Engl J Med. 2015;373:2141–8.

49. Saccone G, Schoen C, Franasiak JM, Scott RT Jr, Berghella V. Supplementation with progestogens in the first trimester of pregnancy to prevent miscarriage in women with unexplained recurrent miscarriage: a systematic review and meta-analysis of randomized, controlled trials. Fertil Steril. 2017;107:430–8.

50. Carp HJ. Progestogens in the prevention of miscarriage. Horm Mol Biol Clin Investig. 2016;27:55–62.

51. Kumar A, Begum N, Prasad S, Aggarwal S, Sharma S. Oral dydrogesterone treatment during early pregnancy to prevent recurrent pregnancy loss and its role in modulation of cytokine production: a double-blind, randomized, parallel, placebo-controlled trial. Fertil Steril. 2014;102:1357–63.

52. Nakagawa K, Kuroda K, Sugiyama R, Yamaguchi K. After 12 consecutive miscarriages, a patient received immunosuppressive treatment and delivered an intact baby. Reprod Med Biol. 2017;16:297–301.

53. Abdolmohammadi-Vahid S, Danaii S, Hamdi K, Jadidi-Niaragh F, Ahmadi M, Yousefi M. Novel immunotherapeutic approaches for treatment of infertility. Biomed Pharmacother. 2016;84:1449–59.

54. Holick MF, Vitamin D. deficiency. N Engl J Med. 2007;357:266–81.

55. Kwak-Kim J, Skariah A, Wu L, Salazar D, Sung N, Ota K. Humoral and cellular autoimmunity in women with recurrent pregnancy losses and repeated implantation failures: a possible role of vitamin D. Autoimmun Rev. 2016;15:943–7.

Chapter 9
Lifestyle Habits and Pregnancy Loss

Keiji Kuroda

Abstract Miscarriage is considered a lifestyle-related disease because the multiple influences of lifestyle habits, including environment and genetics, affect the outcome of pregnancies. Lifestyle-related risk factors for pregnancy loss include smoking, caffeine intake, alcohol consumption, obesity, vitamin D deficiency, and stress. Although it is difficult to determine with accuracy the threshold at which these factors trigger the induction of miscarriage, preconception lifestyle modification for the prevention of pregnancy loss is advisable based on evidence from the literature.

Keywords Pregnancy loss · Recurrent miscarriage · Lifestyle · Smoking · Caffeine · Obesity · Vitamin D · Stress

9.1 Lifestyle Habits

Pregnancy loss occurs in an estimated 10–15% of clinical pregnancies. The risk factors for pregnancy loss are wide variety including thrombophilia, uterine malformation, and thyroid disorders. However, the multiple influences of lifestyle habits such as environment and genetics can affect pregnancy outcomes, and therefore, miscarriage is considered a lifestyle-related disease [1, 2]. Lifestyle habits related to the risk for pregnancy loss include smoking, caffeine intake, alcohol consumption, and obesity. Accurately assessing the threshold at which these factors trigger the induction of miscarriage is difficult. Evidence from the literature suggests that preconception lifestyle modification for the prevention of pregnancy loss is advisable.

K. Kuroda
Center for Reproductive Medicine and Implantation Research, Sugiyama Clinic Shinjuku, Tokyo, Japan

Department of Obstetrics and Gynaecology, Faculty of Medicine, Juntendo University, Tokyo, Japan
e-mail: arthur@juntendo.ac.jp

© Springer Nature Singapore Pte Ltd. 2018
K. Kuroda et al. (eds.), *Treatment Strategy for Unexplained Infertility and Recurrent Miscarriage*, https://doi.org/10.1007/978-981-10-8690-8_9

9.1.1 Smoking

Smoking has adverse effects on pregnancy and neonatal outcomes, including ecto-pic pregnancy, fetal growth restriction, preterm birth, stillbirth, and sudden infant death syndrome [3]. Tobacco smoke contains a complex mixture of toxic chemicals, and nicotine easily crosses the placenta and reaches the fetus [4]. Thus, smoking cessation is recommended for every pregnant woman. A multivariate analysis of potential risk factors in pregnancy loss showed that maternal smoking is strongly associated with an increased risk of early pregnancy loss (odds ratio [OR] 2.00; 95% confidence interval [CI] 1.27–3.15) [5].

Venners et al. reported that paternal tobacco use is also related to early pregnancy loss via passive smoking [6]. The ORs of early pregnancy loss in groups of women who live with partners who smoke fewer than 20 and 20 or more cigarettes daily were 1.04 (95% CI, 0.67–1.63) and 1.81 (95% CI, 1.00–3.29), respectively. Heavy paternal smoking also increases the risk of pregnancy loss. Although cigarette smoking is not a proven risk factor for recurrent miscarriage (RM), the relation between smoking and poor obstetric outcomes has been confirmed. Couples with RM must be informed about the adverse effects of smoking on the likelihood of live birth, and smoking cessation before pregnancy should be recommended.

9.1.2 Caffeine Intake

Caffeine is a natural compound with stimulant effects commonly found in coffee and tea. Klebanoff et al. reported an association between serum levels of the caf-feine metabolite, paraxanthine before pregnancy, and subsequent pregnancy out-comes [7]. Compared with serum paraxanthine levels in controls, those in women whose pregnancies ended in spontaneous miscarriage were higher ($p < 0.001$). Chen et al. reviewed the relationship between caffeine consumption and pregnancy loss in 130,456 women (Fig. 9.1) [8] and found that compared with the risk in pregnant women with no or very low caffeine intake, the relative risk (RR) of pregnancy loss was 1.02 in women with low caffeine intake (50–149 mg/day), 1.16 for moderate intake (150–349 mg/day), 1.40 for high intake (350–699 mg/day), and 1.72 for very high intake ($\geq$700 mg/day). The risk of pregnancy loss related to caffeine intake increased dose dependently (7% higher risk of miscarriage per 100 mg/day of intake).

Moreover, Stefanidou et al. showed that compared with women with <150 mg/day of caffeine intake, women with unexplained RM who had caffeine intakes of 151–300 mg/day and >300 mg/day had ORs for miscarriage of 3.05 (95% CI, 1.24–7.29, $p = 0.012$) and 16.11 (95% CI, 6.55–39.62, $p < 0.001$), respectively [9].

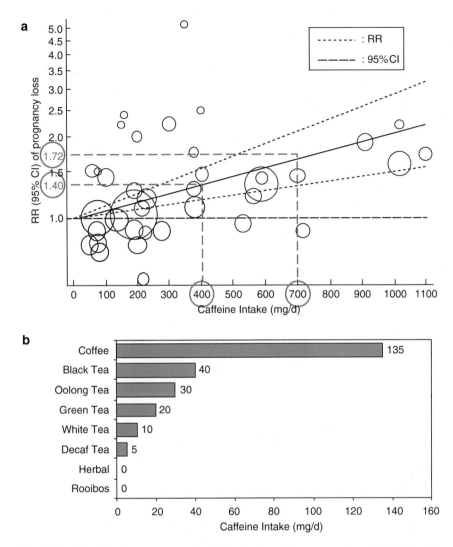

Fig. 9.1 Relationship between maternal caffeine intake and pregnancy loss. (**a**) Relationships between maternal caffeine intake and pregnancy loss reported in various studies. The open circles represent the effect estimates of caffeine intake on pregnancy loss from each study. The circle size indicates the proportional precision of the estimate values. Compared with the risk of pregnancy loss associated with no or very low caffeine intake, the relative risk (RR) of pregnancy loss is reported to be 1.40 for high intake (350–699 mg/day) and 1.72 for very high intake (≥700 mg/day). The risk of pregnancy loss related to caffeine increases dose dependently. *CI* confidence interval. (Chen LW, et al., Public Health Nutr. 2016). (**b**) Average amount of caffeine per serving. The amount of caffeine in three to five cups of coffee exceeds 400 mg, and the RR of pregnancy loss is 1.5–2.0

However, another study showed that caffeine consumption does not increase the risk of RM [10]. Thus, the relationship between caffeine intake and RM remains unclear.

9.1.3 Alcohol Consumption

Maternal heavy alcohol intake during pregnancy is involved in adverse impact on fetus such as malformations (fetal alcohol syndrome), mental retardation, as well as damage of central nervous system (fetal alcohol spectrum disorders) [11]. A safe amount of alcohol intake during pregnancy is still controversial. Kesmodel et al. showed the relationship between the amount of alcohol consumption and pregnancy loss in 24,679 singleton pregnancies [12] and demonstrated that compared with women with one time or less per week of drink, the RRs of spontaneous pregnancy loss in the first trimester were 1.3 (95% CI, 0.8–2.0) for 1–2 drinks per week, 0.8 (95% CI, 0.4–1.7) for 3–4 drinks per week, and 3.7 (95% CI, 2.0–6.8) for 5 or more drinks per week. Harlap et al. surveyed 32,019 pregnant women by questionnaire for drinking [13]. Compared to women without drinking, the survey results showed that RRs of pregnancy losses in the second trimester (15–27 weeks of gestation) were 1.03 (no significant difference), 1.98 ($p < 0.01$), and 3.53 ($p < 0.01$) for pregnant women with less than 1, 1–2, and ≥3 drinks daily. Maconochie et al. also reported a case-control study of 603 women whose last pregnancy had ended in pregnancy loss in the first trimester and 6116 women whose last pregnancy had maintained beyond 12 weeks [14]. ORs of pregnancy losses were 1.46 (95% CI, 1.16–1.85) for drinking regularly at least once a week and 1.64 (95% CI, 1.09–2.47) for drinking more than 14 units (140 ml of pure alcohol, roughly 3500 ml of beer) of alcohol per week. Although no proper study of the adverse effect of consuming alcohol on RM, limitation or cessation of alcohol intake is important for women with a history of RM.

9.1.4 Obesity

Obesity has a significant adverse effect on female fecundity and is associated with infertility, pregnancy loss, and obstetric complications [15]. The World Health Organization defines a body mass index (BMI) of ≥25 kg/m^2 as overweight and a BMI of ≥30 kg/m^2 as obesity. A systematic review reported that compared with the miscarriage rate of women with normal BMIs (10.7%), that in obese women (13.6%) was significantly higher (OR, 1.31, 95% CI, 1.18–1.46) [16]. Obese women also have a prevalence of RM that is significantly higher than that in nonobese women (0.4% versus 0.1%, respectively, OR, 3.51, 95% CI, 1.03–12.01) [16].

It remains unknown whether the increased risk of pregnancy loss in obese women results from decreased endometrial receptivity or low oocyte quality. Outcomes of egg donation programs have demonstrated that miscarriage is mainly caused by endometrial factors [17, 18], and Boots et al. reported that obese women with RM had a rate of euploid miscarriage higher than that of nonobese women (58% versus 37%, respectively; RR, 1.63, 95% CI, 1.08–2.47). The results of these studies suggest that the adverse effects of obesity on the endometrium contribute to pregnancy loss [19]. Basic research has also demonstrated that impaired endometrial function in obese women leads to pregnancy loss [20, 21].

No appropriate study of the effect of weight loss on RM has been performed. However, weight loss improves endocrine profiles and reproductive outcomes, including spontaneous ovulation and the pregnancy rate after infertility treatment [22]. Couples with RM should be informed that maternal obesity is associated with obstetric complications including miscarriage and could have an adverse impact on general health as well as the likelihood of a live birth.

9.1.5 Vitamin D Deficiency

Although the relationship between nutritional complements and pregnancy complications remains controversial, it is reasonable to expect that well-balanced nutritional intake is important for improvement of pregnancy outcomes. Recent reports have shown that vitamin D (VD) deficiency is strongly associated with reproductive failure, including implantation failure after in vitro fertilization and pregnancy complications such as miscarriage, preeclampsia, and gestational diabetes mellitus [23, 24]. VD is a liposoluble vitamin associated with calcium homeostasis. VD also regulates immune functions such as the production of T-helper (Th) cells in a variety of organ systems [25]; therefore, VD deficiency is linked to autoimmune diseases including type 1 diabetes, systemic lupus erythematosus, and autoimmune thyroid disease [26–29].

Hou et al. examined serum levels of the storage form of VD, 25-hydroxyvitamin D_3 (25(OH)VD), and 25-hydroxyvitamin D-1α-hydroxylase (CYP27B1), which catalyzes the activation of 25(OH)VD, in four groups: nulliparous women at 7–9 weeks of gestation who ultimately had (1) successful clinical pregnancies or (2) pregnancy loss and preconception women who ultimately had (3) successful clinical pregnancies or (4) one or more spontaneous first-trimester miscarriages (Fig. 9.2) [30]. Both the pregnant and nonpregnant women with successful pregnancies (groups a and c) had 25(OH)VD and CYP27B1 levels that were significantly higher than those in the women who experienced pregnancy loss (groups b and d) (both $p < 0.01$). Moreover, 96.7% of the preconception women with pregnancy loss had below 30 ng/ml as normal 25(OH)VD levels. Furthermore, Ota et al. reported that compared with RM patients with normal VD levels, RM patients with VD deficiency had higher risks for autoimmune and cellular immune abnormalities in antinuclear antigen antibody, antiphospholipid antibody, thyroperoxidase antibody, and natural killer cell cytotoxicity [31].

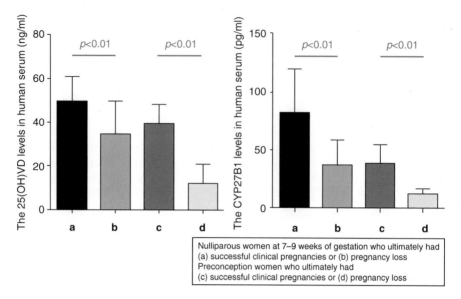

Fig. 9.2 Comparison of pregnant and nonpregnant women who ultimately had successful pregnancies and miscarriages. A study compared serum concentrations of 25-hydroxyvitamin D_3 (25(4)VD) and 25-hydroxyvitamin D-1α-hydroxylase (CYP27B1) in four groups: nulliparous women at 7–9 weeks of gestation who ultimately had (**a**) successful clinical pregnancies or (**b**) pregnancy loss and preconception women who ultimately had (**c**) successful clinical pregnancies or (**d**) one or more spontaneous first-trimester miscarriages (Hou W, et al., Eur J Clin Nutr. 2016)

The impact of VD deficiency and VD supplementation on pregnancy loss remains to be elucidated, but VD may play a key role in regulating maternal immune tolerance for successful pregnancy. The effect of VD supplementation in RM patients with VD deficiency warrants further study.

9.2   Stress

Although clinical pregnancy loss is a common disorder, it is a significant medical event for each patient. In particular, patients with a history of RM feel a roller coaster of emotions between the joy of pregnancy and the grief of losing a child. The repeated experience of pregnancy loss and stillbirth often induces feelings of despair, self-dispraise, and impotence, which lead to depression, anxiety disorders, and insomnia. Indeed, approximately 50% of women who have an abortion experience psychological manifestations such as depression or anxiety in the weeks and months after pregnancy loss [32]. Furthermore, most women with a history of RM become anxious during subsequent pregnancies [33]. Craig et al. reported that in 81 women with RM, 33% were diagnosed with depression, including 7.4% with severe depression [34].

Maternal stress is associated with an increased risk of pregnancy loss [35, 36]. Studies in mice have also shown that stress induces pregnancy loss [37, 38]. In a study of women who miscarried during the first trimester, decidual tissue from subjects with high stress scores had significantly higher numbers of tryptase-positive mast cells, CD8-positive T cells, and tumor necrosis factor-α–positive cells, which suggests that stress triggers the induction of maternal immunological fetal rejection via the activation of cytotoxic T lymphocytes and Th1 cells in the local decidua [39]. Moreover, an elevated maternal cortisol level during early pregnancy is a risk factor for miscarriage [40], and compared with patients without mental health problems, those with any mental health disorder before pregnancy have a significantly higher risk of miscarriage or stillbirth [41]. Contradictory studies have reported no evidence for as a risk factor for abortion [42, 43]; therefore, the adverse effect of stress on pregnancy remains controversial.

Meanwhile the decrease in pregnancy loss rate by mental care after abortion as "tender loving care" was reported [44, 45]. Notably, however, there is no specific remedy for unexplained RM. Trials of patients with unexplained RM who are treated with placebo have shown high live birth rates [46–50] (for details, refer to the section "Past Pilot Study of Unexplained Recurrent Miscarriage"). The administration of a placebo may reduce stress in patients with unexplained RM, thereby lowering pregnancy loss rates. However, the lack of specific risk factors for miscarriage is a cause of further anxiety in patients with RM, which leads to a vicious cycle of pregnancy loss. Some RM patients undergoing treatment describe their uncertainty about subsequent pregnancies as a feeling of entering a dark tunnel. Therefore, it is important for caregivers to inform patients that 75% of women with unexplained RM achieve a live birth after proper evaluation and treatment [44, 51]. The reduced fecundity and increased miscarriage rates associated with advanced reproductive age should be considered. Thus, in patients with diminished ovarian reserves or age >40 years, infertility treatment including in vitro fertilization should be considered even if spontaneous conception has occurred.

References

1. Parazzini F, Bocciolone L, Fedele L, Negri E, La Vecchia C, Acaia B. Risk factors for spontaneous abortion. Int J Epidemiol. 1991;20:157–61.
2. Rai R, Regan L. Recurrent miscarriage. Lancet. 2006;368:601–11.
3. Leung LW, Davies GA. Smoking cessation strategies in pregnancy. J Obstet Gynaecol Can. 2015;37:791–7.
4. Lambers DS, Clark KE. The maternal and fetal physiologic effects of nicotine. Semin Perinatol. 1996;20:115–26.
5. Winter E, Wang J, Davies MJ, Norman R. Early pregnancy loss following assisted reproductive technology treatment. Hum Reprod. 2002;17:3220–3.
6. Venners SA, Wang X, Chen C, Wang L, Chen D, Guang W, Huang A, Ryan L, O'Connor J, Lasley B, Overstreet J, Wilcox A, Xu X. Paternal smoking and pregnancy loss: a prospective study using a biomarker of pregnancy. Am J Epidemiol. 2004;159:993–1001.

7. Klebanoff MA, Levine RJ, DerSimonian R, Clemens JD, Wilkins DG. Maternal serum paraxanthine, a caffeine metabolite, and the risk of spontaneous abortion. N Engl J Med. 1999;341:1639–44.
8. Chen LW, Wu Y, Neelakantan N, Chong MF, Pan A, van Dam RM. Maternal caffeine intake during pregnancy and risk of pregnancy loss: a categorical and dose-response meta-analysis of prospective studies. Public Health Nutr. 2016;19:1233–44.
9. Stefanidou EM, Caramellino L, Patriarca A, Menato G. Maternal caffeine consumption and sine causa recurrent miscarriage. Eur J Obstet Gynecol Reprod Biol. 2011;158:220–4.
10. Zhang BY, Wei YS, Niu JM, Li Y, Miao ZL, Wang ZN. Risk factors for unexplained recurrent spontaneous abortion in a population from southern China. Int J Gynaecol Obstet. 2010;108:135–8.
11. Streissguth AP, O'Malley K. Neuropsychiatric implications and long-term consequences of fetal alcohol spectrum disorders. Semin Clin Neuropsychiatry. 2000;5:177–90.
12. Kesmodel U, Wisborg K, Olsen SF, Henriksen TB, Secher NJ. Moderate alcohol intake in pregnancy and the risk of spontaneous abortion. Alcohol Alcohol. 2002;37:87–92.
13. Harlap S, Shiono PH. Alcohol, smoking, and incidence of spontaneous abortions in the first and second trimester. Lancet. 1980;2:173–6.
14. Maconochie N, Doyle P, Prior S, Simmons R. Risk factors for first trimester miscarriage - results from a UK-population-based case-control study. BJOG. 2007;114:170–86.
15. Metwally M, Ledger WL, Li TC. Reproductive endocrinology and clinical aspects of obesity in women. Ann N Y Acad Sci. 2008;1127:140–6.
16. Boots C, Stephenson MD. Does obesity increase the risk of miscarriage in spontaneous conception: a systematic review. Semin Reprod Med. 2011;29:507–13.
17. Bellver J, Rossal LP, Bosch E, Zuniga A, Corona JT, Melendez F, Gomez E, Simon C, Remohi J, Pellicer A. Obesity and the risk of spontaneous abortion after oocyte donation. Fertil Steril. 2003;79:1136–40.
18. Bellver J, Melo MA, Bosch E, Serra V, Remohi J, Pellicer A. Obesity and poor reproductive outcome: the potential role of the endometrium. Fertil Steril. 2007;88:446–51.
19. Boots CE, Bernardi LA, Stephenson MD. Frequency of euploid miscarriage is increased in obese women with recurrent early pregnancy loss. Fertil Steril. 2014;102:455–9.
20. Metwally M, Tuckerman EM, Laird SM, Ledger WL, Li TC. Impact of high body mass index on endometrial morphology and function in the peri-implantation period in women with recurrent miscarriage. Reprod Biomed Online. 2007;14:328–34.
21. Murakami K, Bhandari H, Lucas ES, Takeda S, Gargett CE, Quenby S, Brosens JJ, Tan BK. Deficiency in clonogenic endometrial mesenchymal stem cells in obese women with reproductive failure – a pilot study. PLoS One. 2013;8:e82582.
22. Farquhar CM, Gillett WR. Prioritising for fertility treatments – should a high BMI exclude treatment? BJOG. 2006;113:1107–9.
23. Zhang MX, Pan GT, Guo JF, Li BY, Qin LQ, Zhang ZL. Vitamin D deficiency increases the risk of gestational diabetes mellitus: a meta-analysis of observational studies. Forum Nutr. 2015;7:8366–75.
24. Mirzakhani H, Litonjua AA, McElrath TF, O'Connor G, Lee-Parritz A, Iverson R, Macones G, Strunk RC, Bacharier LB, Zeiger R, Hollis BW, Handy DE, Sharma A, Laranjo N, Carey V, Qiu W, Santolini M, Liu S, Chhabra D, Enquobahrie DA, Williams MA, Loscalzo J, Weiss ST. Early pregnancy vitamin D status and risk of preeclampsia. J Clin Invest. 2016;126:4702–15.
25. Holick MF. Vitamin D deficiency. N Engl J Med. 2007;357:266–81.
26. Bizzaro G, Shoenfeld Y. Vitamin D and autoimmune thyroid diseases: facts and unresolved questions. Immunol Res. 2015;61:46–52.
27. El-Fakhri N, McDevitt H, Shaikh MG, Halsey C, Ahmed SF. Vitamin D and its effects on glucose homeostasis, cardiovascular function and immune function. Horm Res Paediatr. 2014;81:363–78.
28. Terrier B, Derian N, Schoindre Y, Chaara W, Geri G, Zahr N, Mariampillai K, Rosenzwajg M, Carpentier W, Musset L, Piette JC, Six A, Klatzmann D, Saadoun D, Patrice C, Costedoat-

Chalumeau N. Restoration of regulatory and effector T cell balance and B cell homeostasis in systemic lupus erythematosus patients through vitamin D supplementation. Arthritis Res Ther. 2012;14:R221.

29. Di Filippo P, Scaparrotta A, Rapino D, Cingolani A, Attanasi M, Petrosino MI, Chuang K, Di Pillo S, Chiarelli F. Vitamin D supplementation modulates the immune system and improves atopic dermatitis in children. Int Arch Allergy Immunol. 2015;166:91–6.

30. Hou W, Yan XT, Bai CM, Zhang XW, Hui LY, Yu XW. Decreased serum vitamin D levels in early spontaneous pregnancy loss. Eur J Clin Nutr. 2016;70:1004–8.

31. Ota K, Dambaeva S, Han AR, Beaman K, Gilman-Sachs A, Kwak-Kim J. Vitamin D deficiency may be a risk factor for recurrent pregnancy losses by increasing cellular immunity and autoimmunity. Hum Reprod. 2014;29:208–19.

32. Lok IH, Neugebauer R. Psychological morbidity following miscarriage. Best Pract Res Clin Obstet Gynaecol. 2007;21:229–47.

33. Kolte AM, Olsen LR, Mikkelsen EM, Christiansen OB, Nielsen HS. Depression and emotional stress is highly prevalent among women with recurrent pregnancy loss. Hum Reprod. 2015;30:777–82.

34. Craig M, Tata P, Regan L. Psychiatric morbidity among patients with recurrent miscarriage. J Psychosom Obstet Gynaecol. 2002;23:157–64.

35. Li W, Newell-Price J, Jones GL, Ledger WL, Li TC. Relationship between psychological stress and recurrent miscarriage. Reprod Biomed Online. 2012;25:180–9.

36. Sugiura-Ogasawara M, Furukawa TA, Nakano Y, Hori S, Aoki K, Kitamura T. Depression as a potential causal factor in subsequent miscarriage in recurrent spontaneous aborters. Hum Reprod. 2002;17:2580–4.

37. Arck PC, Merali FS, Stanisz AM, Stead RH, Chaouat G, Manuel J, Clark DA. Stress-induced murine abortion associated with substance P-dependent alteration in cytokines in maternal uterine decidua. Biol Reprod. 1995;53:814–9.

38. Arck PC, Merali F, Chaouat G, Clark DA. Inhibition of immunoprotective CD8+ T cells as a basis for stress-triggered substance P-mediated abortion in mice. Cell Immunol. 1996;171:226–30.

39. Arck PC, Rose M, Hertwig K, Hagen E, Hildebrandt M, Klapp BF. Stress and immune mediators in miscarriage. Hum Reprod. 2001;16:1505–11.

40. Nepomnaschy PA, Welch KB, McConnell DS, Low BS, Strassmann BI, England BG. Cortisol levels and very early pregnancy loss in humans. Proc Natl Acad Sci U S A. 2006;103:3938–42.

41. Gold KJ, Dalton VK, Schwenk TL, Hayward RA. What causes pregnancy loss? Preexisting mental illness as an independent risk factor. Gen Hosp Psychiatry. 2007;29:207–13.

42. Nelson DB, McMahon K, Joffe M, Brensinger C. The effect of depressive symptoms and optimism on the risk of spontaneous abortion among inner city women. J Womens Health (Larchmt). 2003;12:569–76.

43. Plana-Ripoll O, Parner E, Olsen J, Li J. Severe stress following bereavement during pregnancy and risk of pregnancy loss: results from a population-based cohort study. J Epidemiol Community Health. 2016;70:424–9.

44. Clifford K, Rai R, Regan L. Future pregnancy outcome in unexplained recurrent first trimester miscarriage. Hum Reprod. 1997;12:387–9.

45. Stray-Pedersen B, Stray-Pedersen S. Etiologic factors and subsequent reproductive performance in 195 couples with a prior history of habitual abortion. Am J Obstet Gynecol. 1984;148:140–6.

46. Schleussner E, Kamin G, Seliger G, Rogenhofer N, Ebner S, Toth B, Schenk M, Henes M, Bohlmann MK, Fischer T, Brosteanu O, Bauersachs R, Petroff D, Grp E. Low-molecular-weight heparin for women with unexplained recurrent pregnancy loss a multicenter trial with a minimization randomization scheme. Ann Intern Med. 2015;162:601–U193.

47. Tang AW, Alfirevic Z, Turner MA, Drury J, Topping J, Dawood F, Farquharson R, Quenby S. A pilot, double blind randomised controlled trial of prednisolone for women with recurrent miscarriage and raised uterine natural killer cell density. Hum Reprod. 2011;26:268–1161.

48. Coomarasamy A, Williams H, Truchanowicz E, Seed PT, Small R, Quenby S, Gupta P, Dawood F, Koot YEM, Atik RB, Bloemenkamp KWM, Brady R, Briley AL, Cavallaro R, Cheong YC, Chu JJ, Eapen A, Ewies A, Hoek A, Kaaijk EM, Koks CAM, Li TC, MacLean M, Mol BW, Moore J, Ross JA, Sharpe L, Stewart J, Vaithilingam N, Farquharson RG, Kilby MD, Khalaf Y, Goddijn M, Regan L, Rai R. A randomized trial of progesterone in women with recurrent miscarriages. N Engl J Med. 2015;373:2141–8.
49. Pasquier E, de Saint Martin L, Bohec C, Chauleur C, Bretelle F, Marhic G, Le Gal G, Debarge V, Lecomte F, Denoual-Ziad C, Lejeune-Saada V, Douvier S, Heisert M, Mottier D. Enoxaparin for prevention of unexplained recurrent miscarriage: a multicenter randomized double-blind placebo-controlled trial. Blood. 2015;125:2200–5.
50. Wong LF, Porter TF, Scott JR. Immunotherapy for recurrent miscarriage. Cochrane Database Syst Rev. 2014;10:CD000112.
51. Brigham SA, Conlon C, Farquharson RG. A longitudinal study of pregnancy outcome following idiopathic recurrent miscarriage. Hum Reprod. 1999;14:2868–71.

Chapter 10
Perturbation of Endometrial Decidualization

Keisuke Murakami, Keiji Kuroda, and Jan J. Brosens

Abstract The hallmark of the reproductive system in women is cyclic decidualization and menstruation. In contrast to other mammals, decidualization of the human endometrium is initiated by endocrine, rather than embryonic, cues. Decidual response is induced by the postovulatory rise in progesterone and local cyclic AMP production. Endometrial shedding in menstruation is triggered by falling progesterone levels, and then endometrium initiates the next regenerative process. Adequate interactions between a developmentally competent embryo and a receptive decidualized endometrium are indispensable for reproductive success. Emerging evidences suggest that decidualizing cells act as a biosensor for embryo quality upon implantation and determine whether to support further development or trigger early rejection. Further, recent findings focus on the role of endometrial MSCs in organizing endometrial regeneration and decidualization. Here, we provide an overview of decidualization and then expand to clinical reflections for recurrent pregnancy loss and recurrent implantation failure.

10.1 Introduction

Reproduction in humans is remarkably inefficient compared to many other species. Monthly fecundity rates (MFR) in fertile couples average only 20% [1]. In contrast, MFR of other mammals such as rabbit and baboon are approximately 80–90%. The

K. Murakami
Department of Obstetrics and Gynaecology, Juntendo University Faculty of Medicine, Tokyo, Japan

K. Kuroda (✉)
Center for Reproductive Medicine and Implantation Research, Sugiyama Clinic Shinjuku, Tokyo, Japan

Department of Obstetrics and Gynaecology, Faculty of Medicine, Juntendo University, Tokyo, Japan
e-mail: arthur@juntendo.ac.jp

J. J. Brosens
The Division of Biomedical Sciences, Clinical Science Research Laboratories, Warwick Medical School, Coventry, UK

© Springer Nature Singapore Pte Ltd. 2018
K. Kuroda et al. (eds.), *Treatment Strategy for Unexplained Infertility and Recurrent Miscarriage*, https://doi.org/10.1007/978-981-10-8690-8_10

reasons for the inefficient human reproduction system may be multifactorial, but it is primarily attributed to the high prevalence of chromosomal abnormalities in embryos lowering their developmental potential. Recent array-based technology revealed that the frequency and complexity of chromosomal abnormalities in human preimplantation embryos are much higher than previously thought [2, 3]. Mertzanidou et al. reported that chromosomal aberrations were detected in over 70% of good-quality cleavage stage IVF embryos [4]. The reason for the genomic instability of human preimplantation embryos has not been clarified. However, emerging evidence suggests that the human endometrium plays an active and important role controlling implanting embryos [5, 6].

The hallmark of the human reproductive cycle is cyclic decidualization and menstruation triggered by endocrine, rather than embryonic, cues [5]. Increasing evidence has clarified that decidualizing cells act as a biosensor for embryo quality upon implantation [5–8]. Adequate interactions between a developmentally competent embryo and a receptive decidualized endometrium are a key step for successful implantation and subsequent pregnancy maintenance. Failure to express the receptive phenotype in the endometrium is responsible for subfertility and implantation failure, whereas prolonged excessive endometrial receptivity permits implantation of delayed or compromised embryos resulting in early pregnancy loss [9]. In this section, we provide an overview of decidualization and then expand to clinical implications including implantation failure and early pregnancy loss.

10.2 Overview of Endometrial Regeneration and Decidualization

The human endometrium undergoes more than 400 menstrual cycles during a period of woman's reproductive years. This dynamic menstrual cycle is divided into three phases: menstruation, proliferative, and secretory (Fig. 10.1). Menstruation is the first phase of the uterine menstrual cycle and stimulates cyclical endometrial regeneration through the recruitment and activation of endometrial mesenchymal stem cells (MSCs). The endometrium initiates proliferation with gradually increasing amount of estrogen. After ovulation, increasing progesterone produced by the corpus luteum and local cyclic AMP production stimulates the endometrial differentiation process known as decidualization [5]. This process is initiated around the terminal spiral arteries and morphologically characterized by transformation of stromal fibroblasts into specialized secretory decidual cells. From a functional perspective, decidualization has the important roles of regulating trophoblast invasion, mobilizing specialized uterine natural killer (uNK) cells, and controlling unique vascular remodeling. As decidualization progresses, endometrial stromal cells transition through two distinct functional phenotypes: an initial acute inflammatory state followed by an anti-inflammatory, mature secretory state.

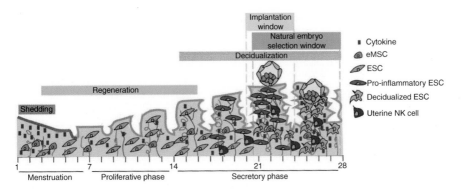

Fig. 10.1 Cyclical endometrial regeneration and decidualization. During each cycle, the human endometrium undergoes regenerative process characterized by shedding, proliferation, and differentiation. Abundant cytokines produced by the endometrium during menstruation recruit and activate endometrial mesenchymal stem cells and induce cyclical regeneration. Upon decidualization, the human endometrium becomes receptive to the implanting embryo; this period is the implantation window. As decidualization progresses, endometrial stromal cells transition from an acute inflammatory state to an anti-inflammatory, mature secretory state. Decidualized endometrial cells have a role in detecting embryo quality and determining whether to support further development or trigger disposal of the implanting embryo. Identification of an abnormal embryo results in rejection with endometrial shedding in menstruation, which then initiates the next regenerative process. *eMSC* endometrial mesenchymal stem cell, *ESC* endometrial stromal cell

This dynamic inflammatory secretome switch in decidualization coincides with the window of implantation and natural embryo selection.

10.3 Implantation Window

Implantation is a complex process characterized by the acceptance of a semialloge-neic embryo by the maternal endometrium. Adequate interactions between a developmentally competent embryo and a receptive decidualized endometrium are indispensable for successful implantation. The process of implantation is subdivided into several phases: apposition, adhesion, penetration, and trophoblast invasion. These sequential complex steps can be successfully accomplished during only a self-limited period known as the implantation window [10]. This brief period coincides with days 20–24 of the menstrual cycle, thus 6–10 days after the luteinizing hormone surge [5, 11]. Previously, Wilcox et al. studied the relationship between the time of implantation and the pregnancy outcome by measuring daily urinary ovarian hormone metabolites and hCG from fertile couples who conceived naturally [12]. In this study, 84% of conceptions could be detected between 8 and 10 days after ovulation. Early pregnancy loss was least frequent when implantation occurred between 6 and 9 days (13 early losses among 102 pregnancies, 13%), and the risk rose to 26% with implantation on day 10, 52% on day 11, and 82% after day 11 [12]. The timing of implantation is a significant contributing factor for successful pregnancy.

10.4 Natural Embryo Selection

Recent evidence suggests that decidualizing endometrial stromal cells serve as bio-sensor for embryo quality upon implantation [5–8]. This observation introduced the concept of "natural embryo selection," which means that decidualizing endometrial cells respond to individual preimplantation embryos in a manner that either supports further development or facilitates early rejection [5, 6]. Teklenburg et al. used a human co-culture model consisting of decidualizing endometrial stromal cells and single-hatched blastocysts to identify the soluble factors involved in implantation [7]. In this study, the co-culture with a normally developing blastocyst had no significant effect on the secretion of implantation factors by decidualizing stromal cells. However, a remarkable response was noted when the embryo seemed to be arrested during the co-culture period, characterized by selective inhibition of several interleukins, C-C motif chemokine 11 (CCL11), and heparin-binding EGF-like growth factor (HB-EGF) secretion. Co-cultures were performed in the same way with undifferentiated endometrial stromal cells, but the distinct response was not noted, irrespective of embryo quality [7]. Weimar et al. employed a modified migration assay, consisting of a monolayer of decidualizing human endometrial stromal cells with a single human embryo placed in the migratory zone [8]. Decidualizing cells could selectively migrate toward high-grade, but not low-grade, human embryos [8]. In the process of acquiring the role of biosensor for implanting embryos, human endometrial stromal cells need to appropriately adapt and rebalance their receptivity versus selectivity traits for successful implantation. A prolonged or excessive receptive phenotype could facilitate implantation of even compromised embryos, thus increasing the likelihood of miscarriage. In contrast, expressing an excessively selective phenotype could reject even the developmentally competent embryos, thus leading to implantation failure and conception delay (Fig. 10.2) [5].

10.5 Decidualization and Recurrent Pregnancy Loss

Approximately 15% of clinically confirmed pregnancies result in miscarriage. Most miscarriages are sporadic and caused by chromosomal aberrations of the conceptus. However, some couples experience early pregnancy loss repeatedly, and they are considered to have a distinct disorder. The American Society for Reproductive Medicine defines recurrent pregnancy loss (RPL) as two or more pregnancy losses, whereas the European Society for Human Reproduction and Embryology has adopted a definition of three or more consecutive pregnancy failures [13, 14]. It is estimated that approximately 5% of women suffer two consecutive miscarriages, and 1% of women suffer three or more consecutive miscarriages [15]. Ogasawara et al. reported that, with each additional miscarriage, the frequency of abnormal embryonic karyotypes decreases, whereas the likelihood of subsequent miscarriage increases [16]. Known risk factors for RPL include parental chromosomal,

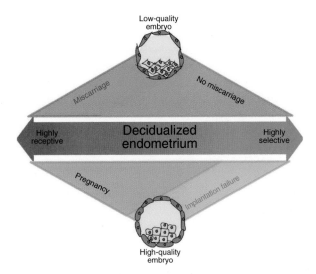

Fig. 10.2 Balancing endometrial receptivity and selectivity. Human preimplantation embryos are genomically remarkably diverse. To achieve reproductive success, the human endometrium needs to adapt and rebalance its receptivity and selectivity. An excessively receptive endometrium could facilitate implantation of even compromised embryos, thus increasing the likelihood of miscarriage. In contrast, an excessively selective endometrium could reject even developmentally competent embryos, leading to implantation failure and conception delay. Referred from Gellersen et al. [5], partially modified

immunological, thrombophilic, endocrine, and uterine anatomical abnormalities. However, in over 50% of RPL cases, no specific cause is identified even after detailed examinations [17]. Furthermore, most perceived causes of RPL lack specificity and are also commonly present in women with normal pregnancies. It is suggested that some women may suffer RPL due to a super-receptive endometrium that permits implantation of even compromised embryos [9]. MFRs of super-fertile women are 60% or more, which is remarkably higher than normal fertile (20%) and subfertile (5%) women [9]. It is estimated that 79% of women are fertile, 18% subfertile, and 3% super-fertile [18]. A retrospective woman-based analysis of the time-to-pregnancy (TTP) intervals in 560 RPL couples revealed that 40% could be considered super-fertile, defined by a mean TTP of 3 months or less [18]. Fortunately, the cumulative live birth rate after several miscarriages is still predicted to be high in most RPL couples, which implies the decidual response is programmed to vary in each cycle and adequate embryo-endometrial interactions can still occur for a successful pregnancy [5]. Previous in vitro assays demonstrated that human endometrial stromal cells from RPL women shows abnormal decidual responses characterized by a prolonged proinflammatory response, inadequate induction of decidual marker genes, increased vulnerability to oxidative stress, aberrant responses to hCG, and inability to distinguish between high- and low-quality human embryos [5]. Although the underlying mechanisms of decidualization remain incompletely understood, recent findings focus on the role of endometrial MSCs in organizing endometrial regeneration and decidualization [19]. It seems plausible to hypothesize that the responsiveness of endometrial cells to decidual signals in each cycle relates to the precedent activation of regenerative MSCs. Recently, it was reported that MSCs are localized to the endometrial perivascular microenvironment and establish distinct cytokine and chemokine profiles in the decidual process. This implies a potential role in regulating trophoblast invasion and governing local immune responses [19]. Further, intriguing findings suggest that there is an inverse correlation between the abundance of clonogenic MSCs in the endometrium and the number of previous miscarriages [20]. These findings encourage the development of novel treatment strategies targeting MSCs in recurrent pregnancy loss, although further studies are expected.

10.6 Decidualization and Recurrent Implantation Failure

Implantation is the key rate-limiting step in assisted reproductive technology (ART). In ART, failed implantation is defined as the lack of an hCG rise to detectable levels after embryo transfer. Recurrent implantation failure (RIF) is defined as the absence of implantation following consecutive transfers of high-quality embryos. The 2005 ESHRE PGD Consortium defines RIF as the absence of implantation after three or more embryo transfers with high-quality embryos or after replacement of a total of ten or more embryos in multiple transfers, with the exact number to be determined by each center [21]. The cause of failed implantation can be iatrogenic, lie with the embryo, the maternal uterine environment, or a combination. Maternal uterine factors can be subdivided into anatomical and non-anatomical disorders. Anatomical disorders include submucosal myoma, endometrial polyps, and uterine malformation. If these disorders are detected by screening, they can be treated using surgical intervention. Non-anatomical disorders include perturbation of decidualization, mismatched implantation window, abnormal local immune surveillance, and chronic endometritis. Decidualization is characterized by transition from the acute inflammatory to anti-inflammatory phase. The initial acute inflammatory phase renders the endometrium receptive for implantation, whereas the following mature secretory phenotype enables the endometrium to select embryos and maintain pregnancy [22]. Recent secretome analysis of primary endometrial stromal cells isolated prior to successful or failed IVF cycles revealed that secretome profiles diverge between both groups [23]. Contrary to RPL, some RIF women may have an aberrant highly selective mechanism that inappropriately rejects good-quality embryos [9].

10.7 Treatment Strategies

10.7.1 Progesterone Treatment in Early Pregnancy

Progesterone is an indispensable female sex hormone that induces decidualization and is essential for successful implantation and pregnancy maintenance. Some women may suffer RPL or RIF because of inadequate progesterone secretion and/

or impaired responsiveness of endometrial cells to progesterone actions. Therefore, supplementation with progesterone can be beneficial, although not always. Kumar et al. conducted a double blind, placebo-controlled, randomized trial with oral dydrogesterone administration in unexplained RPL women and demonstrated a reduction in the incidence of subsequent miscarriages compared to placebo [24]. In contrast, a recent multicenter, double blind, placebo-controlled, randomized trial investigating the effectiveness of vaginal progesterone administration in unexplained RPL women showed no improvement in live birth rate [25], perhaps reflecting the fact that progesterone treatment was initiated only when the pregnancy was well established. A recent meta-analysis of randomized, controlled trials showed that supplementation with progestogens reduces the risk of subsequent miscarriage (RR 0.72, 95% CI 0.53–0.97) and increases the live birth rate (RR 1.07, 95% CI 1.02–1.15) compared to the placebo group [26]. There are discrepancies regarding the effectiveness of progesterone in RPL women depending on the study quality and differences in route, dosage, and period of progesterone administration. Taken together, progesterone administration to enhance decidualization remains a reasonable treatment option for unexplained recurrent reproductive failures, although further trials are warranted.

10.7.2 Endometrial Scratching for Impaired Decidualization and RIF

The effectiveness of artificial endometrial injury to improve subsequent decidual responses has been long recognized. Indeed, many clinical studies demonstrated the benefits of endometrial scratching in the luteal phase prior to an IVF/ICSI cycle for increasing implantation and pregnancy rates. Karimzadeh et al. conducted a randomized controlled trial investigating the effectiveness of endometrial scratching performed during the previous cycle in patients with RIF and showed that implantation and clinical pregnancy rates increase after endometrial scratching [27]. In contrast, a randomized controlled trial of 300 unselected subfertile women failed to show a beneficial effect of endometrial scratch, performed in the preceding cycle, on improving the ongoing pregnancy rate [28]. These conflicting results may be attributable to patient differences, such as the number of previous failed implantations. So far, no trial has been performed in RPL women. The mechanism to improve endometrial receptivity by artificial scratching has not been incompletely understood; however, cytokines, chemokines, and growth factors produced by locally injured endometrium are presumed to be key factors for improving subsequent pregnancy rates. Liang et al. compared the secretome profile between endometrial injury and non-endometrial injury groups, and they showed that endometrial injury promoted the induction of several cytokines including IFN-γ and VEGF and improved clinical pregnancy rates [29]. MSCs that possess the homing ability to the injury sites might be key regulators for promoting endometrial regeneration and providing a suitable microenvironment for implantation. Whether recruitment and activation of endometrial MSCs account for the improvement of endometrial performance following artificial tissue injury remains to be tested.

10.7.3 Prednisolone Treatment for RPL

RPL is considered a multifactorial disorder, and an aberrant immunological response to pregnancy is thought to play a major role in the pathogenesis. Several studies have demonstrated the association between RPL and the high density of uNK cells in the preimplantation endometrium [30–32]. Quenby et al. have demonstrated that the increased density of uNK cells associated with the aberrant angiogenesis might expose the embryo to excessive oxidative stress, thus increasing the risk of miscarriage [33]. They have also demonstrated that high number of uNK cell in preimplantation endometrium of recurrent miscarriage women can be efficiently reduced by administration of prednisolone [34]. However, a pilot randomized controlled trial that recruited 40 recurrent miscarriage women with high uNK cell density showed that prednisolone administration had no significant improvement in live birth rate (RR 1.5, 95% CI 0.79–2.86) [35]. To date, the effectiveness of prednisolone remains controversial. An excessive anti-inflammatory effect by prednisolone could also raise the adverse concern inhibiting implantation; prednisolone administration is not recommended for unselected recurrent miscarriage women.

References

1. Evers JL. Female subfertility. Lancet. 2002;360(9327):151–9.
2. Ledbetter DH. Chaos in the embryo. Nat Med. 2009;15(5):577–83.
3. Vanneste E, Voet T, Le Caignec C, Ampe M, Konings P, et al. Chromosome instability is common in human cleavage-stage embryos. Nat Med. 2009;15(5):577–83.
4. Mertzanidou A, Wilton L, Cheng J, Spits C, Vanneste E, et al. Microarray analysis reveals abnormal chromosomal complements in over 70% of 14 normally developing human embryos. Hum Reprod. 2013;28(1):256–64.
5. Gellersen B, Brosens JJ. Cyclic decidualization of the human endometrium in reproductive health and failure. Endocr Rev. 2014;35(6):851–905.
6. Brosens JJ, Salker MS, Teklenburg G, Nautiyal J, Salter S, et al. Uterine selection of human embryos at implantation. Sci Rep. 2014;4:3894.
7. Teklenburg G, Salker M, Molokhia M, Lavery S, Trew G, et al. Natural selection of human embryos: decidualizing endometrial stromal cells serve as sensors of embryo quality upon implantation. PLoS One. 2010;5(4):e10258.
8. Weimar CH, Kavelaars A, Brosens JJ, Gellersen B, de Vreeden-Elbertse JM, et al. Endometrial stromal cells of women with recurrent miscarriage fail to discriminate between high- and low-quality human embryos. PLoS One. 2012;7(7):e41424.
9. Teklenburg G, Salker M, Heijnen C, Macklon NS, Brosens JJ. The molecular basis of recurrent pregnancy loss: impaired natural embryo selection. Mol Hum Reprod. 2010;16(12):886–95.
10. van Mourik MS, Macklon NS, Heijnen CJ. Embryonic implantation: cytokines, adhesion molecules, and immune cells in establishing an implantation environment. J Leukoc Biol. 2009;85(1):4–19.
11. Bergh PA, Navot D. The impact of embryonic development and endometrial maturity on the timing of implantation. Fertil Steril. 1992;58(3):537–42.
12. Wilcox AJ, Baird DD, Weinberg CR. Time of implantation of the conceptus and loss of pregnancy. N Engl J Med. 1999;340(23):1796–9.

13. Practice Committee of American Society for Reproductive Medicine. Definitions of infertility and recurrent pregnancy loss: a committee opinion. Fertil Steril. 2013;99(1):63.
14. Jauniaux E, Farquharson RG, Christiansen OB, Exalto N. Evidence-based guidelines for the investigation and medical treatment of recurrent miscarriage. Hum Reprod. 2006;21(9):2216–22.
15. Sugiura-Ogasawara M, Suzuki S, Ozaki Y, Katano K, Suzumori N, et al. Frequency of recurrent spontaneous abortion and its influence on further marital relationship and illness: the Okazaki cohort study in Japan. J Obstet Gynaecol Res. 2013;39(1):126–31.
16. Ogasawara M, Aoki K, Okada S, Suzumori K. Embryonic karyotype of abortuses in relation to the number of previous miscarriages. Fertil Steril. 2000;73(2):300–4.
17. Branch DW, Gibson M, Silver RM. Clinical practice. Recurrent miscarriage. N Engl J Med. 2010;363(18):1740–7.
18. Salker M, Teklenburg G, Molokhia M, Lavery S, Trew G, et al. Natural selection of human embryos: impaired decidualization of endometrium disables embryo-maternal interactions and causes recurrent pregnancy loss. PLoS One. 2010;5(4):e10287.
19. Murakami K, Lee YH, Lucas ES, Chan YW, Durairaj RP, et al. Decidualization induces a secretome switch in perivascular niche cells of the human endometrium. Endocrinology. 2014;155(11):4542–53.
20. Lucas ES, Dyer NP, Murakami K, Lee YH, Chan YW, et al. Loss of endometrial plasticity in recurrent pregnancy loss. Stem Cells. 2016;34(2):346–56.
21. Thornhill AR, de Die-Smulders CE, Geraedts JP, Harper JC, Harton GL, et al. ESHRE PGD Consortium. ESHRE PGD Consortium 'Best practice guidelines for clinical preimplantation genetic diagnosis (PGD) and preimplantation genetic screening (PGS)'. Hum Reprod. 2005;20(1):35–48.
22. Salker MS, Nautiyal J, Steel JH, Webster Z, Sućurović S, et al. Disordered IL-33/ST2 activation in decidualizing stromal cells prolongs uterine receptivity in women with recurrent pregnancy loss. PLoS One. 2012;7(12):e52252.
23. Peter Durairaj RR, Aberkane A, Polanski L, Maruyama Y, Baumgarten M, et al. Deregulation of the endometrial stromal cell secretome precedes embryo implantation failure. Mol Hum Reprod. 2017. https://doi.org/10.1093/molehr/gax023. [Epub ahead of print]
24. Kumar A, Begum N, Prasad S, Aggarwal S, Sharma S. Oral dydrogesterone treatment during early pregnancy to prevent recurrent pregnancy loss and its role in modulation of cytokine production: a double-blind, randomized, parallel, placebo-controlled trial. Fertil Steril. 2014;102(5):1357–63.
25. Coomarasamy A, Williams H, Truchanowicz E, Seed PT, Small R, et al. A randomized trial of progesterone in women with recurrent miscarriages. N Engl J Med. 2015;373(22):2141–8.
26. Saccone G, Schoen C, Franasiak JM, Scott RT Jr, Berghella V. Supplementation with progestogens in the first trimester of pregnancy to prevent miscarriage in women with unexplained recurrent miscarriage: a systematic review and meta-analysis of randomized, controlled trials. Fertil Steril. 2017;107(2):430–8.
27. Karimzadeh MA, Ayazi Rozbahani M, Tabibnejad N. Endometrial local injury improves the pregnancy rate among recurrent implantation failure patients undergoing in vitro fertilisation/intra cytoplasmic sperm injection: a randomised clinical trial. Aust N Z J Obstet Gynaecol. 2009;49(6):677–80.
28. Yeung TW, Chai J, Li RH, Lee VC, Ho PC, et al. The effect of endometrial injury on ongoing pregnancy rate in unselected subfertile women undergoing in vitro fertilization: a randomized controlled trial. Hum Reprod. 2014;29(11):2474–81.
29. Liang Y, Han J, Jia C, Ma Y, Lan Y, et al. Effect of endometrial injury on secretion of endometrial cytokines and IVF outcomes in women with unexplained subfertility. Mediators Inflamm. 2015;2015:757184.
30. Quenby S, Bates M, Doig T, Brewster J, Lewis-Jones DI, et al. Pre-implantation endometrial leukocytes in women with recurrent miscarriage. Hum Reprod. 1999;14(9):2386–91.

31. Clifford K, Flanagan AM, Regan L. Endometrial CD56+ natural killer cells in women with recurrent miscarriage: a histomorphometric study. Hum Reprod. 1999;14(11):2727–30.
32. Tuckerman E, Laird SM, Prakash A, Li TC. Prognostic value of the measurement of uterine natural killer cells in the endometrium of women with recurrent miscarriage. Hum Reprod. 2007;22(8):2208–13.
33. Quenby S, Nik H, Innes B, Lash G, Turner M, et al. Uterine natural killer cells and angiogenesis in recurrent reproductive failure. Hum Reprod. 2009;24(1):45–54.
34. Quenby S, Kalumbi C, Bates M, Farquharson R, Vince G. Prednisolone reduces preconceptual endometrial natural killer cells in women with recurrent miscarriage. Fertil Steril. 2005;84(4):980–4.
35. Tang AW, Alfirevic Z, Turner MA, Drury JA, Small R, et al. A feasibility trial of screening women with idiopathic recurrent miscarriage for high uterine natural killer cell density and randomizing to prednisolone or placebo when pregnant. Hum Reprod. 2013;28(7):1743–52.

Chapter 11
Treatment Strategy for Unexplained Recurrent Miscarriage

Keiji Kuroda

Abstract Couples with unexplained recurrent miscarriage (RM) cannot achieve live birth, because of repeated sporadic abortion or undetected causes of RM on common examinations. The undetected causes of RM include complexed multiple risk factors of pregnancy loss as multifactorial disease and perturbation of endometrial decidualization. To avoid subsequent pregnancy loss, recommendations for RM treatment include modification of lifestyle habits to eliminate risk factors of miscarriage; vitamin D supplementation, if deficient; adequate diagnosis and treatment of chronic endometritis; and oral dydrogesterone treatment as a part of "tender loving care." If patients have diminished ovarian reserves or are >40 years old, infertility treatment should be recommended. If subsequent pregnancy ends in miscarriage, chromosome analysis of chorionic villi samplings is required for planning treatment strategy of the subsequent pregnancy. If the result is euploid, further investigations for the cause of RM and reexamination of treatment strategy are required.

Keywords Unexplained recurrent miscarriage · Decidualization · Dydrogesterone Vitamin D · Tender loving care · Chromosome analysis of chorionic villi

11.1 Screening for Recurrent Miscarriage (RM) and Lifestyle Modification

In humans, miscarriage accounts for 10–15% of all clinical pregnancies. RM is defined as three or more consecutive miscarriages detected in the intrauterine cavity [1]. The incidences of two or three consecutive accidental miscarriages occur at calculated rates of 1–3% and 0.1–0.3%, respectively. These incidence

K. Kuroda
Center for Reproductive Medicine and Implantation Research, Sugiyama Clinic Shinjuku, Tokyo, Japan

Department of Obstetrics and Gynaecology, Faculty of Medicine, Juntendo University, Tokyo, Japan
e-mail: arthur@juntendo.ac.jp

© Springer Nature Singapore Pte Ltd. 2018
K. Kuroda et al. (eds.), *Treatment Strategy for Unexplained Infertility and Recurrent Miscarriage*, https://doi.org/10.1007/978-981-10-8690-8_11

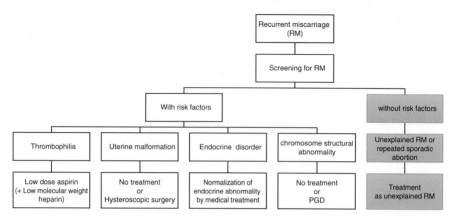

Fig. 11.1 Treatment protocol of recurrent miscarriage (RM). Risk factors for RM include thrombophilia, uterine malformation, endocrine abnormality, and chromosome abnormality. A basic remedy for RM is a therapeutic strategy against the causes of pregnancy losses. When no risk factor was found by common RM screening, couples should be treated as having unexplained RM with undetected factors. PGD and preimplantation genetic diagnosis

rates are significantly low compared with the actual prevalence rates of 4.2% and 0.9%, respectively [2]. Therefore, screening for RM is important when planning treatment. Risk factors for RM include thrombophilia, uterine malformation, endocrine abnormality, and chromosome structural abnormality (for details, refer to the section entitled "Unexplained recurrent miscarriage-Introduction"). A general treatment protocol for RM is shown in Fig. 11.1. The treatment methods for RM with risk factors are omitted. When focusing on unexplained RM, patients may suffer repeated sporadic abortions fortuitously. However, some couples cannot achieve live birth because of factors undetected by common RM screening methods. The undetected causes of RM include complexed multiple risk factors of pregnancy loss as multifactorial disease and perturbation of endometrial decidualization.

Miscarriage is considered a lifestyle-related disease, because multiple factors of lifestyle habits, such as environment and genetics, can impact pregnancy outcomes [3, 4]. Therefore, an interview with the patients to ask their lifestyle habits and psychological trauma from a previous pregnancy is very important when planning the treatment strategy for a subsequent pregnancy. Risk factors of lifestyle habits for miscarriage are shown in Fig. 11.2. Factors that increase risks of miscarriage 1.5- to 2-fold include maternal as well as paternal smoking of >10–20 cigarettes per day [5, 6], caffeine intake of >2–3 cups of coffee per day [7], alcohol consumption of >2 drinks per week [8], and obesity (body mass index >30 kg/m^2) [9]. These lifestyle habits are associated with early sporadic miscarriage. However, the linkage between RM and each individual factor remains controversial. Multifactorial combinations may trigger repetitive pregnancy losses. Therefore, adverse lifestyle factors should be modified for next pregnancy, such as cessation of smoking and alcohol intake, reduction of caffeine intake, and weight loss by exercise.

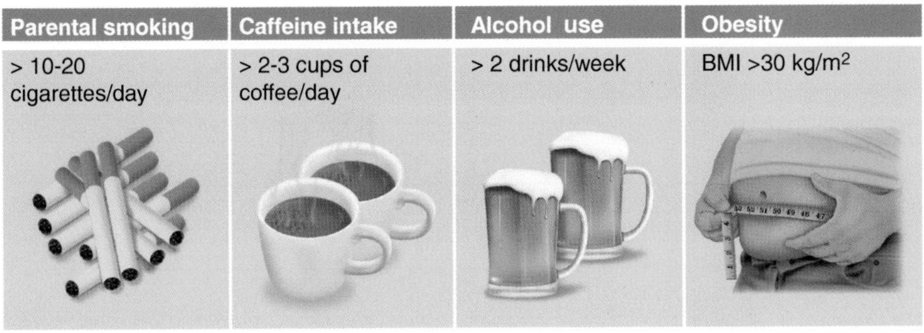

Parental smoking	Caffeine intake	Alcohol use	Obesity
> 10-20 cigarettes/day	> 2-3 cups of coffee/day	> 2 drinks/week	BMI >30 kg/m²

Fig. 11.2 Risks for miscarriage increase 1.5- to 2-fold according to lifestyle habits. Risk factors of lifestyle habits causing sporadic miscarriage are shown. The risks that increase miscarriage by 1.5- to 2-fold are maternal as well as paternal smoking of >10–20 cigarettes per day, caffeine intake of >2–3 cups of coffee per day, alcohol consumption of >2 drinks per week, and obesity (body mass index >30 kg/m²)

Vitamin D deficiency is also associated with pregnancy loss [10]. Confirmation of serum 25-hydroxyvitamin D_3 [25(OH)VD] level and preconception vitamin D supplementation are also important to prevent pregnancy loss. Further, maternal stress is related to an increased risk of pregnancy loss [11, 12]. Most women with a history of repeated pregnancy losses and stillbirth have suffered physical and psychological stress and have experienced anxiety for a subsequent pregnancy [13]. Therefore, it is important to inform patients that 75% of women with unexplained RM achieve a live birth after proper evaluation and treatment to relieve their stress and to support them with periodic consultation as tender loving care [14, 15] (for details, refer to the section entitled "Unexplained recurrent miscarriage-Lifestyle habits and pregnancy loss").

11.2 Advanced Maternal Age and Miscarriage

In developed countries, there is a concern about change in the population structure, such as late reproductive age of women resulting in a declining fertility rate. A large-scale study of 634,272 Danish women and 1,221,546 pregnancies showed that the risk of a spontaneous pregnancy loss was 11.1, 11.9, 15.0, 24.6, 51.0, and 93.4% in those aged 20–24, 25–29, 30–34, 35–39, 40–44, and ≥45 years, respectively. The incidence of spontaneous pregnancy loss increases exponentially with maternal age in women aged ≥35 years (Fig. 11.3) [16]. Therefore, consideration of the patient's age is important for a successful live birth when treating for RM.

In women with RM aged ≤30 years at the first consultation, the cumulative live birth rate reaches >80% in 5 years; in fact, pregnancy outcome is little affected by aging. However, the cumulative live birth rate in women with RM is approximately 70%, 60%, and only 40% in those aged 30–34, 35–39, and ≥40 years, respectively (Fig. 11.4) [17]. Therefore, patients aged ≥40 years with unexplained RM should be persuaded to consider infertility treatment, even if they have conceived spontaneously.

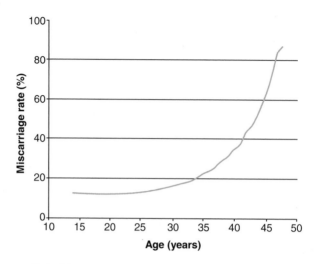

Fig. 11.3 Age-specific incidence rates of miscarriage. A large-scale study in Denmark showed that the risks of a spontaneous pregnancy loss in women aged 20–24, 25–29, 30–34, 35–39, 40–44, and ≥45 years were 11.1%, 11.9%, 15.0%, 24.6%, 51.0%, and 93.4%, respectively. The incidence of spontaneous pregnancy loss increases exponentially with maternal age in women aged ≥35 years. Nybo Andersen AM et al. BMJ, 2000

11.3 Impaired Decidualization of Endometrium and RM

Fertility can be assessed by the monthly fecundity rate (MFR), i.e., the probability of achieving pregnancy within one menstrual cycle. Compared with other mammalian species, the average human MFR is relatively low at 20%. In 1950, Tietze et al. [18] reported that 79% of 1727 women who desired pregnancy had normal fertility, whereas 18% were subfertile or infertile, and 3% were superfertile with a MFR of ≥60%. In humans, the incidence of embryo wastage and miscarriage is estimated to be 30% before implantation and 30% before 6 weeks of gestation, and 10–20% of clinical pregnancies are classified as "embryo wastage iceberg" (Fig. 11.5). Recent reports demonstrated that decidualized endometrial stromal cells serve as biosensors of embryo quality [19–21]. The endometrial cells in superfertile women may have disordered embryo receptive ability (natural embryo selection hypothesis; Fig. 11.5). RM partially occurs due to inadequate endometrial receptivity of preimplantation embryos, which should have been wasted as in superfertility [22]. The incidence of early pregnancy loss increases with later implantation periods after ovulation in an exponential manner (Fig. 11.6) [23]. Some patients with unexplained RM may repeat pregnancy losses with a delayed window of implantation due to impaired decidualization of the endometrium.

During the postovulatory period, the uterine endometrium is decidualized under the effect of progesterone. Endometrial angiogenesis is induced to receive

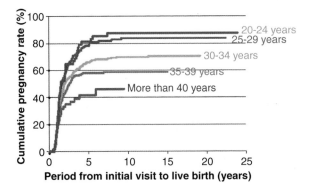

Fig. 11.4 Age-specific cumulative pregnancy rate of women with a history of recurrent miscarriage (RM). In women with RM aged ≤30 years at the first consultation, the cumulative live birth rate reached >80% in 5 years. However, the cumulative live birth rate in women with RM aged 30–34, 35–39, and ≥40 years was approximately 70%, 60%, and only 40%, respectively. Lund M et al., Obstet Gynecol, 2012

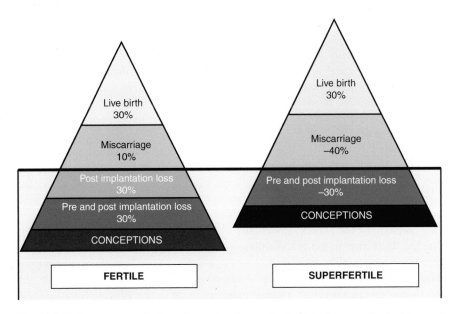

Fig. 11.5 Embryo wastage iceberg (natural embryo selection). In humans, the incidence of embryo wastage is estimated to be 30% before implantation and 30% before 6 weeks of gestation, and 10–20% of clinical pregnancies are classified as "embryo wastage iceberg." Superfertile woman with extremely high fecundity and miscarriage rates was reported in 3% of women. The endometrial cells in superfertile women may have disordered embryo receptive ability (natural embryo selection hypothesis). Repeated pregnancy losses occur partially due to inadequate endometrial receptivity of preimplantation embryos, which should have been wasted in superfertility. Teklenburg G et al., Mol Hum Reprod, 2010

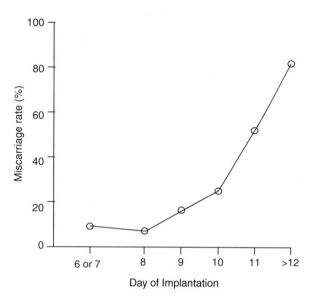

Fig. 11.6 Timing of implantation and miscarriage. The relationship between timing of implantation and pregnancy loss after natural conception is shown. The incidence of early pregnancy loss increases with later implantation period after ovulation in an exponential manner. Wilcox AJ et al., N Engl J Med, 1999

a competent embryo by angiogenic factors, including inflammatory cytokines secreted from uterine natural killer (uNK) cells [24]. uNK cells also play a significant role in spiral artery remodeling and trophoblast invasion during early pregnancy [25]. uNK cells, which are CD56^{bright} and CD16$^-$, have low cellular cytotoxicity and are phenotypically and functionally different from CD56^{dim} and CD16$^+$ peripheral blood NK cells. Several publications have reported a relationship between RM and aberrant high uNK cell density in mid-luteal phase endometrial cells [26–28]. Glucocorticoids, such as prednisolone, can suppress excess numbers of uNK cells and abnormal angiogenesis [29, 30]. Therefore, successful live births in patients with RM with abnormally high levels of uNK cells after prednisolone treatment have been reported [29]. Tang et al. [31] performed a pilot randomized controlled trial of prednisolone treatment (20 mg for 6 weeks, 10 mg for 1 week, 5 mg for 1 week) for women with RM with a high density of uNK cells. The live birth rate in the prednisolone group was higher at 60.0% (12/20 cases) compared with 40.0% (8/20 cases) in the placebo group, yet there was no significant difference. Regarding implantation, an inflammatory response with pro-inflammatory cytokines and prostaglandins is an important process for an embryo to attach and invade into the decidual endometrium [32–34]. Glucocorticoids may potentially inhibit implantation.

Another player, progesterone, is an essential factor for decidualization of the endometrium, implantation, and maintenance of pregnancy. Progesterone is also an activator of local cortisone during decidual transformation of the endometrium leading to direct and indirect regulation of uNK cell density via glucocorticoid receptors [28, 35, 36]. Furthermore, progesterone can inhibit contraction of uterine smooth muscle and production of prostaglandins, and it also induces production of helper T-cell cytokines, leading to optimization of immune tolerance for an embryo [37]. Therefore, progesterone is expected to be therapeutically efficacious for RM. Coomarasamy et al. [38] reported a multicenter, randomized controlled trial (PROMISE study) of vaginal progesterone suppositories (400 mg twice daily) for women with unexplained RM. Of 836 women with three or more prior miscarriages, the live birth rate in the progesterone group was 65.8% (262/398 cases), which was comparable to the 63.3% (271/428 cases) rate in the placebo group. Synthetic progestogen, including dydrogesterone, is effective for unexplained RM, according to a systematic review [39, 40]. In particular, Kumar et al. [41] demonstrated the impact of dydrogesterone treatment (10 mg twice daily) on unexplained RM via regulation of helper T-cell cytokines. Therefore, systemic administration of synthetic progestogen may be effective compared with vaginal natural progesterone treatment. Also, progesterone treatment has no harmful effects on implantation, placentation, and the fetus (for details, refer to the section entitled "Unexplained recurrent miscarriage-Perturbation of endometrial decidualization" and "Past pilot studies for unexplained recurrent miscarriage").

Chronic endometritis (CE), which is a persistent inflammation of the uterine endometrium, occurs in approximately 50–70% of women with RM [42, 43]. CE is caused by a wide variety of microorganisms [44]; thus, broad-spectrum antibiotics against a wide range of bacteria, such as oral doxycycline or ciprofloxacin + metronidazole, are the most common treatment for CE [45]. CE is also a cause of impaired endometrial decidualization [46]. Although we cannot identify whether CE results in or from miscarriage, CE is strongly associated with infertility and pregnancy loss. Therefore, CE should be diagnosed and adequately treated before initiation of therapy for subsequent pregnancy (for details, refer to the section entitled "Unexplained infertility-Implantation failure 1: intrauterine circumstance and embryo–endometrium synchrony").

11.4 Treatment Strategy for Unexplained RM

To our knowledge, there is no established efficient treatment for unexplained RM according to past pilot studies. However, combined various treatments and supplementations may prevent pregnancy loss. The treatment protocol for unexplained RM is shown in Fig. 11.7. First, we can confirm intrauterine circumstances using hysteroscopy and serum storage form of vitamin D [25(OH)VD] and treat patients, if any problems are detected. Tender loving care is also an important therapy for relieving stress and anxiety. If some treatments are to be used as placebo for

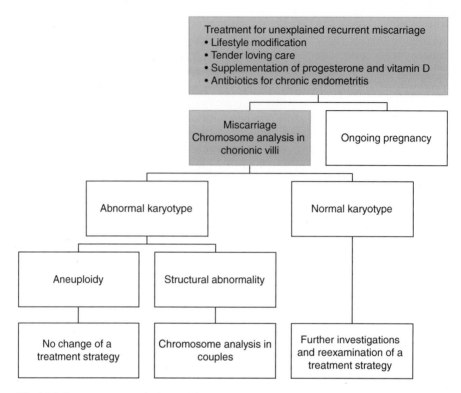

Fig. 11.7 Treatment protocol of unexplained recurrent miscarriage (RM). For avoidance of subsequent pregnancy loss, recommendations for a RM treatment strategy include modification of lifestyle habits to eliminate risk factors of miscarriage, vitamin D supplementation, if deficient, adequate diagnosis and treatment of chronic endometritis, and oral dydrogesterone treatment as a part of tender loving care. When subsequent pregnancy ended in miscarriage, chromosome analysis in chorionic villi samplings was required to plan treatment strategy of the subsequent pregnancy. When the analysis of villi showed chromosomal aneuploidy, miscarriage was unavoidable. Therefore, current treatment should be continued. When structural chromosomal abnormality was found, parental genetic analysis was needed. If the result was euploid, further investigations for the cause of RM and reexamination of a treatment strategy are required

psychological support, oral dydrogesterone supplementation is recommended because it is harmless for implantation and pregnancy and effective for optimization of endometrial decidualization. Low-dose aspirin and prednisolone treatment have anti-inflammatory actions that may have adverse impacts on implantation. Also, if the patients have diminished ovarian reserve or are >40 years old, infertility treatment including in vitro fertilization should be recommended even if spontaneous pregnancy has occurred.

In patients with RM in whom subsequent pregnancy unfortunately ended in miscarriage despite every possible treatment, when planning the treatment strategy for the subsequent pregnancy, it is necessary to clarify whether the RM resulted from maternal or fetal problems. Chromosome analysis of chorionic villi samplings is the only alternative to determine the answer. When obtaining chorionic villi samplings, accurate separation of chorionic villi from maternal decidua is crucial for successful analysis of the miscarriage tissue. The villi appear white and fluffy after washing with normal saline solution. Murugappan et al. [47] demonstrated a video of the separation technique of villi. When analysis of the villi showed chromosomal aneuploidy, miscarriage was unavoidable without preimplantation genetic screening. Therefore, current treatment should be continued for the subsequent pregnancy. When a structural chromosomal abnormality was found, parental genetic analysis was required. If parental chromosomal abnormalities were recognized, the subsequent pregnancy loss rate was higher than that in couples with normal karyotypes. When proceeding to preimplantation genetic diagnosis for avoiding pregnancy losses, the cumulative live birth rate is comparable to that of natural conception [48]. Therefore, it is important for gynecologists to inform patients that 63–66% of couples with chromosomal abnormalities can achieve live birth after spontaneous conception [48–50]. If the result of chromosomal analysis of pregnancy tissue is euploid, further investigations for the cause of RM and reexamination of a treatment strategy are required.

References

1. Jauniaux E, Farquharson RG, Christiansen OB, Exalto N. Evidence-based guidelines for the investigation and medical treatment of recurrent miscarriage. Hum Reprod. 2006;21:2216–22.
2. Sugiura-Ogasawara M, Suzuki S, Ozaki Y, Katano K, Suzumori N, Kitaori T. Frequency of recurrent spontaneous abortion and its influence on further marital relationship and illness: the Okazaki cohort study in Japan. J Obstet Gynaecol Res. 2013;39:126–31.
3. Parazzini F, Bocciolone L, Fedele L, Negri E, La Vecchia C, Acaia B. Risk factors for spontaneous abortion. Int J Epidemiol. 1991;20:157–61.
4. Rai R, Regan L. Recurrent miscarriage. Lancet. 2006;368:601–11.
5. Winter E, Wang J, Davies MJ, Norman R. Early pregnancy loss following assisted reproductive technology treatment. Hum Reprod. 2002;17:3220–3.
6. Venners SA, Wang X, Chen C, Wang L, Chen D, Guang W, Huang A, Ryan L, O'Connor J, Lasley B, Overstreet J, Wilcox A, Xu X. Paternal smoking and pregnancy loss: a prospective study using a biomarker of pregnancy. Am J Epidemiol. 2004;159:993–1001.
7. Chen LW, Wu Y, Neelakantan N, Chong MF, Pan A, van Dam RM. Maternal caffeine intake during pregnancy and risk of pregnancy loss: a categorical and dose-response meta-analysis of prospective studies. Public Health Nutr. 2016;19:1233–44.
8. Kesmodel U, Wisborg K, Olsen SF, Henriksen TB, Secher NJ. Moderate alcohol intake in pregnancy and the risk of spontaneous abortion. Alcohol Alcohol. 2002;37:87–92.
9. Boots CE, Bernardi LA, Stephenson MD. Frequency of euploid miscarriage is increased in obese women with recurrent early pregnancy loss. Fertil Steril. 2014;102:455–9.
10. Hou W, Yan XT, Bai CM, Zhang XW, Hui LY, Yu XW. Decreased serum vitamin D levels in early spontaneous pregnancy loss. Eur J Clin Nutr. 2016;70:1004–8.
11. Sugiura-Ogasawara M, Furukawa TA, Nakano Y, Hori S, Aoki K, Kitamura T. Depression as a potential causal factor in subsequent miscarriage in recurrent spontaneous aborters. Hum Reprod. 2002;17:2580–4.
12. Li W, Newell-Price J, Jones GL, Ledger WL, Li TC. Relationship between psychological stress and recurrent miscarriage. Reprod Biomed Online. 2012;25:180–9.

13. Lok IH, Neugebauer R. Psychological morbidity following miscarriage. Best Pract Res Clin Obstet Gynaecol. 2007;21:229–47.
14. Clifford K, Rai R, Regan L. Future pregnancy outcome in unexplained recurrent first trimester miscarriage. Hum Reprod. 1997;12:387–9.
15. Brigham SA, Conlon C, Farquharson RG. A longitudinal study of pregnancy outcome following idiopathic recurrent miscarriage. Hum Reprod. 1999;14:2868–71.
16. Nybo Andersen AM, Wohlfahrt J, Christens P, Olsen J, Melbye M. Maternal age and fetal loss: population based register linkage study. BMJ. 2000;320:1708–12.
17. Lund M, Kamper-Jorgensen M, Nielsen HS, Lidegaard O, Andersen AMN, Christiansen OB. Prognosis for live birth in women with recurrent miscarriage. What is the best measure of success? Obstet Gynecol. 2012;119:37–43.
18. Tietze C, Guttmacher AF, Rubin S. Time required for conception in 1727 planned pregnancies. Fertil Steril. 1950;1:338–46.
19. Teklenburg G, Salker M, Molokhia M, Lavery S, Trew G, Aojanepong T, Mardon HJ, Lokugamage AU, Rai R, Landles C, Roelen BAJ, Quenby S, Kuijk EW, Kavelaars A, Heijnen CJ, Regan L, Brosens JJ, Macklon NS. Natural selection of human embryos: decidualizing endometrial stromal cells serve as sensors of embryo quality upon implantation. PLoS One. 2010;5:e10258.
20. Brosens JJ, Salker MS, Teklenburg G, Nautiyal J, Salter S, Lucas ES, Steel JH, Christian M, Chan Y-W, Boomsma CM, Moore JD, Hartshorne GM, Sucurovic S, Mulac-Jericevic B, Heijnen CJ, Quenby S, Koerkamp MJG, Holstege FCP, Shmygol A, Macklon NS. Uterine selection of human embryos at implantation. Sci Rep. 2014;4:3894.
21. Weimar CHE, Kavelaars A, Brosens JJ, Gellersen B, de Vreeden-Elbertse JMT, Heijnen CJ, Macklon NS. Endometrial stromal cells of women with recurrent miscarriage fail to discriminate between high-and low-quality human embryos. PLoS One. 2012;7:e41424.
22. Teklenburg G, Salker M, Heijnen C, Macklon NS, Brosens JJ. The molecular basis of recurrent pregnancy loss: impaired natural embryo selection. Mol Hum Reprod. 2010;16:886–95.
23. Wilcox AJ, Baird DD, Wenberg CR. Time of implantation of the conceptus and loss of pregnancy. N Engl J Med. 1999;340:1796–9.
24. Moffett-King A. Natural killer cells and pregnancy. Nat Rev Immunol. 2002;2:656–63.
25. Hanna J, Goldman-Wohl D, Hamani Y, Avraham I, Greenfield C, Natanson-Yaron S, Prus D, Cohen-Daniel L, Arnon TI, Manaster I, Gazit R, Yutkin V, Benharroch D, Porgador A, Keshet E, Yagel S, Mandelboim O. Decidual NK cells regulate key developmental processes at the human fetal-maternal interface. Nat Med. 2006;12:1065–74.
26. Quenby S, Nik H, Innes B, Lash G, Turner M, Drury J, Bulmer J. Uterine natural killer cells and angiogenesis in recurrent reproductive failure. Hum Reprod. 2009;24:45–54.
27. Clifford K, Flanagan AM, Regan L. Endometrial CD56+natural killer cells in women with recurrent miscarriage: a histomorphometric study. Hum Reprod. 1999;14:2727–30.
28. Kuroda K, Venkatakrishnan R, James S, Sucurovic S, Mulac-Jericevic B, Lucas ES, Takeda S, Shmygol A, Brosens JJ, Quenby S. Elevated periimplantation uterine natural killer cell density in human endometrium is associated with impaired corticosteroid signaling in decidualizing stromal cells. J Clin Endocrinol Metab. 2013;98:4429–37.
29. Quenby S, Kalumbi C, Bates M, Farquharson R, Vince G. Prednisolone reduces preconceptual endometrial natural killer cells in women with recurrent miscarriage. Fertil Steril. 2005;84:980–4.
30. Lash GE, Bulmer JN, Innes BA, Drury JA, Robson SC, Quenby S. Prednisolone treatment reduces endometrial spiral artery development in women with recurrent miscarriage. Angiogenesis. 2011;14:523–32.
31. Tang A-W, Alfirevic Z, Turner MA, Drury J, Quenby S. Prednisolone trial: study protocol for a randomised controlled trial of prednisolone for women with idiopathic recurrent miscarriage and raised levels of uterine natural killer (uNK) cells in the endometrium. Trials. 2009;10:102.
32. Chard T. Cytokines in implantation. Hum Reprod Update. 1995;1:385–96.

33. Sharkey A. Cytokines and implantation. Rev Reprod. 1998;3:52–61.
34. Kelly RW, King AE, Critchley HOD. Cytokine control in human endometrium. Reproduction. 2001;121:3–19.
35. Kuroda K, Venkatakrishnan R, Salker MS, Lucas ES, Shaheen F, Kuroda M, Blanks A, Christian M, Quenby S, Brosens JJ. Induction of 11 beta-HSD 1 and activation of distinct mineralocorticoid receptor- and glucocorticoid receptor-dependent gene networks in decidualizing human endometrial stromal cells. Mol Endocrinol. 2013;27:192–202.
36. Guo W, Li PF, Zhao GF, Fan HY, Hu YL, Hou YY. Glucocorticoid receptor mediates the effect of progesterone on uterine natural killer cells. Am J Reprod Immunol. 2012;67:463–73.
37. Szekeres-Bartho J, Balasch J. Progestagen therapy for recurrent miscarriage. Hum Reprod Update. 2008;14:27–35.
38. Coomarasamy A, Williams H, Truchanowicz E, Seed PT, Small R, Quenby S, Gupta P, Dawood F, Koot YEM, Atik RB, Bloemenkamp KWM, Brady R, Briley AL, Cavallaro R, Cheong YC, Chu JJ, Eapen A, Ewies A, Hoek A, Kaaijk EM, Koks CAM, Li TC, MacLean M, Mol BW, Moore J, Ross JA, Sharpe L, Stewart J, Vaithilingam N, Farquharson RG, Kilby MD, Khalaf Y, Goddijn M, Regan L, Rai R. A randomized trial of progesterone in women with recurrent miscarriages. N Engl J Med. 2015;373:2141–8.
39. Saccone G, Schoen C, Franasiak JM, Scott RT Jr, Berghella V. Supplementation with progestogens in the first trimester of pregnancy to prevent miscarriage in women with unexplained recurrent miscarriage: a systematic review and meta-analysis of randomized, controlled trials. Fertil Steril. 2017;107:430–8.
40. Carp HJ. Progestogens in the prevention of miscarriage. Horm Mol Biol Clin Investig. 2016;27:55–62.
41. Kumar A, Begum N, Prasad S, Aggarwal S, Sharma S. Oral dydrogesterone treatment during early pregnancy to prevent recurrent pregnancy loss and its role in modulation of cytokine production: a double-blind, randomized, parallel, placebo-controlled trial. Fertil Steril. 2014;102:1357–63.
42. Zolghadri J, Momtahan M, Aminian K, Ghaffarpasand F, Tavana Z. The value of hysteroscopy in diagnosis of chronic endometritis in patients with unexplained recurrent spontaneous abortion. Eur J Obstet Gynecol Reprod Biol. 2011;155:217–20.
43. McQueen DB, Perfetto CO, Hazard FK, Lathi RB. Pregnancy outcomes in women with chronic endometritis and recurrent pregnancy loss. Fertil Steril. 2015;104:927–31.
44. Kitaya K, Matsubayashi H, Yamaguchi K, Nishiyama R, Takaya Y, Ishikawa T, Yasuo T, Yamada H. Chronic endometritis: potential cause of infertility and obstetric and neonatal complications. Am J Reprod Immunol. 2016;75:13–22.
45. Johnston-MacAnanny EB, Hartnett J, Engmann LL, Nulsen JC, Sanders MM, Benadiva CA. Chronic endometritis is a frequent finding in women with recurrent implantation failure after in vitro fertilization. Fertil Steril. 2010;93:437–41.
46. Wu D, Kimura F, Zheng L, Ishida M, Niwa Y, Hirata K, Takebayashi A, Takashima A, Takahashi K, Kushima R, Zhang G, Murakami T. Chronic endometritis modifies decidualization in human endometrial stromal cells. Reprod Biol Endocrinol. 2017;15:16.
47. Murugappan G, Gustin S, Lathi RB. Separation of miscarriage tissue from maternal decidua for chromosome analysis. Fertil Steril. 2014;102:e9–e10.
48. Ikuma S, Sato T, Sugiura-Ogasawara M, Nagayoshi M, Tanaka A, Takeda S. Preimplantation genetic diagnosis and natural conception: a comparison of live birth rates in patients with recurrent pregnancy loss associated with translocation. PLoS One. 2015;10:e0129958.
49. Sugiura-Ogasawara M, Aoki K, Fujii T, Fujita T, Kawaguchi R, Maruyama T, Ozawa N, Sugi T, Takeshita T, Saito S. Subsequent pregnancy outcomes in recurrent miscarriage patients with a paternal or maternal carrier of a structural chromosome rearrangement. J Hum Genet. 2008;53:622–8.
50. Flynn H, Yan J, Saravelos SH, Li TC. Comparison of reproductive outcome, including the pattern of loss, between couples with chromosomal abnormalities and those with unexplained repeated miscarriages. J Obstet Gynaecol Res. 2014;40:109–16.

Printed by Printforce, the Netherlands